Healthy Pregnancy

A 15-Minute Quick Guide to Help You Ward off Worries on Your Pregnancy

Karen Kennedy

PUBLISHED BY:
Karen Kennedy
Copyright © 2012

Table of Contents

Introduction.. 7

What Is a Healthy Pregnancy? 7

Tips on How to Remain Healthy during Pregnancy 7

What You Need to Do to Have a Healthy Pregnancy 7

Chapter 1: Preparing for Pregnancy 8

Thing to Consider before Getting Pregnant................................. 8

How to Prepare for Pregnancy 9

Ways to Increase Your Chances of Getting Pregnant..................... 9

Having a Baby Is Literally Good for You 12

When to Start Taking Prenatal Vitamins...................................... 12

Chapter 2: Signs of Pregnancy 12

The Early Signs of Pregnancy... 12

When Do Signs of Pregnancy Typically Start? 14

How to Recognize Signs of Pregnancy.. 14

Taking a Home Pregnancy Test and HCG Levels........................... 15

Choosing an OB/GYN or a Midwife 16

The First Prenatal Appointment: What to Expect......................... 19

Placenta: How It Works.. 20

Danger Signs in Early Pregnancy 21

Chapter 3: Vitamins and Supplements 22

Choosing Your Pregnancy Supplements 22

How Does Folic Acid Support a Healthy Pregnancy?.................... 22

Why Is Iron Important? 23

Benefits of Fish Oil during Pregnancy... 24

The Amount of Vitamins Needed for a Healthy Pregnancy............ 24

Chapter 4: Tests That Can Be Performed during Pregnancy **25**

Types of Tests That Are Routinely Done at the Doctor's Office *25*

Ultrasounds: Why Do Them and What Are They Used for? *27*

When Should I Decline Testing? *28*

Chapter 5: Pregnancy Diet **28**

A Healthy Diet Is Important during Pregnancy *28*

What Are Some Healthy Pregnancy Diets? *28*

Choosing Healthy Snacks *30*

Foods to Avoid while Pregnant *30*

Healthy Pregnancy Eating Habits *31*

How to Control Pregnancy Junk Food Cravings *32*

How Much Water Do You Need? *32*

Chapter 6: Fitness in Pregnancy **33**

How Does Fitness Help You Have a Healthy Pregnancy? *33*

Tips for Healthy Exercise during Pregnancy *33*

How Pregnancy Yoga Helps You Keep Fit and Healthy *33*

What is a Healthy Pregnancy Weight Gain? *33*

How to Not Gain Too Much Weight during Pregnancy *34*

Chapter 7: Sex during Pregnancy **34**

How to Have Sex during Pregnancy *34*

What Are the Benefits of Sex during Pregnancy? *35*

When is Sex Allowed and When Is It Not Allowed? *36*

Chapter 8: Healthy Sleeping in Pregnancy **36**

Sleep during Pregnancy *36*

What Sleeping Positions Are Good during Pregnancy? *36*

Sleeping Better throughout the Pregnancy *37*

Chapter 9: Oral Care during Pregnancy 37

How to Care for Your Teeth during Pregnancy 37

Why Are Your Gums Sensitive During Pregnancy? 38

Bleeding Gums during Pregnancy 38

How Cavities Can Affect Your Pregnancy 38

Chapter 10: Work Meets Pregnancy 39

Working during Pregnancy: Do's and Don'ts 39

What Can You Do to Promote a Healthy Pregnancy at Work? 40

How Does the Stress Level at Your Job Affect a Healthy Pregnancy? 40

Chapter 11: Common Pregnancy Ailments 41

Yeast Infection during Pregnancy 41

Pregnancy Constipation: Are Stool Softeners Safe? 42

How to Have a Healthy Pregnancy with Hypertension 42

How to Prevent Stretch Marks during Pregnancy 43

What Helps to Relieve Swollen Feet during Pregnancy? 44

Tips on How to Relieve Pelvic Pressure during the Last Trimester 45

Chapter 12: Complications That Can Occur 46

What is Gestational Diabetes? 46

What is Fetal Demise? 47

What is Preeclampsia? 49

What Are the Signs of Preeclampsia? 49

Other Complications to Watch For 50

Chapter 13: The Baby inside You 53

What does a Baby Look Like inside the Womb? 53

Can You Reduce Birth Defects? 60

Caution: What You Take May Harm Your Baby 61

How to Ensure Healthy Brain Development of Your Baby during Pregnancy ... 62

Why Do Babies Kick Inside the Womb?..62

Chapter 14: Pre-Delivery: What You Need to Know? 63

Why Would a Childbirth Class Be Helpful?..63

What Types of Childbirth Classes Are There?...63

Why You Should Avoid Unnecessary Medical Interventions 65

How to Create a Birth Plan to Avoid Unnecessary Medical Interventions.........68

What to Buy for Your Baby: The Essentials 70

What You Should Bring to the Hospital or Birthing Center 73

What Items Are Needed for a Home Birth?..77

Identify True Labor Contractions...78

What to Expect during Delivery...79

Introduction

What Is a Healthy Pregnancy?

A healthy pregnancy is a pregnancy that is long, boring, and uneventful. You want that. Healthy pregnancy actually starts before you get pregnant. If you are trying to have a baby, there are things you can do before conception that can help you attain a healthy pregnancy. You can start taking prenatal vitamins, finding the obstetrician/gynecologist (OB/GYN) or midwife you'd like to take care of you, and exercising. All of these things and more can be found in the following chapters.

Tips on How to Remain Healthy during Pregnancy

To remain healthy during pregnancy, you can

- Take vitamins and supplements (Chapter 3)

- Take tests that can catch problems early on (Chapter 4)

- Follow a healthy diet (Chapter 5)

- Exercise (Chapter 6).

All that and more is covered in the following chapters.

What You Need to Do to Have a Healthy Pregnancy

To have a healthy pregnancy, you can start by taking vitamins. It is also important that you stop drinking, smoking and taking drugs before you conceive. Go to your OB/GYN or midwife before you conceive for a pre-conception appointment. If you have a pap-smear due, this would be the perfect time to do it. You can also find out what kind of vitamins to use; your caregiver may even give you a prescription for some. Your caregiver can even go through your current medications and update them with something that is friendlier to a growing baby.

Chapter 1: Preparing for Pregnancy

Thing to Consider before Getting Pregnant

Are you secured financially? Are you healthy? Do you have drug prescriptions that may not be safe for a growing baby? Are you in a healthy relationship?

Financial security is a plus when you decide to expand your family. I don't call it a *must*. If it seems like you will never have a family if you have to wait for financial security, and you are mentally and physically ready for a baby, go for it. It is harder rearing a child if you have little income and no savings, but it isn't impossible. You may have to let go of some luxury purchases and buy non-name brand food, but it can be done. Financial security ensures that you don't have to scrimp and save so often, but many of today's families have children when they are financially secure, and then lose that security when they are laid off. If you are lucky, you'll have family to help you out when you need it. If you are not, there are government programs that may be helpful to you.

Another plus is being healthy already. For me, weight is not an issue, as there are plenty of women who are overweight and still healthy, but a healthy weight before pregnancy is nicer. You can buy cuter maternity clothes if you are not too overweight, and you are more noticeably pregnant to the people around you. However, if you have high blood pressure, diabetes, or other conditions, you may have a harder pregnancy than most. Most blood pressure medications cannot be taken during pregnancy. Some can, so ask your caregiver before you conceive—or as soon as you find out you are pregnant.

It is also important to review your relationship. Do you fight often? Do you think that having a baby will make everything better than it is? Does your significant other belittle you, hit you, or cheat on you? If you answered yes to any of these questions, it isn't the right time for you to conceive a child. Remember, you are bringing an innocent new life into the equation. If you don't feel safe, your child won't feel safe.

This is one of the questions your caregiver or midwife will ask you when you go in for your first appointment. They ask for the sake of the child, but also for you. You cannot have a healthy pregnancy if you are often stressed, hurt, or scared.

How to Prepare for Pregnancy

To start preparing for pregnancy, schedule consultation appointments with multiple caregivers or midwives to find a caregiver that is one you feel safe and comfortable with (see Choosing an OB/GYN or a Midwife). Take a daily prenatal vitamin, eat healthy meals, and exercise. If you are a smoker, quit. If you drink often, stop. If you partake in illegal drugs, don't. If you are taking prescription medications, consult with your caregiver to find a medication that is not harmful to a growing baby. Either start exercising or continue exercising. Your caregiver will let you know if and when you need to change your exercise routine.

Ways to Increase Your Chances of Getting Pregnant

There are many ways to increase your chances of getting pregnant. If you don't want to make a business out of it, just have sex around the time you think you may ovulate. However, if you don't know when you ovulate, there are many ways to find out when you are ready to.

Ovulation prediction kits (OPKs), which are available for purchase online and at your local grocery store, can increase your chances of conceiving. Many of the companies who produce pregnancy tests now produce OPKs. Some are harder to read than others, so find the one that is right for you. What an OPK does is detect your luteal surge. There are three phases in your cycle. These phases correspond with the different hormones produced at certain times. The first phase begins when you start menstruating—the very first day of menstruation—this is a small phase called the follicular phase. The second phase is the ovulatory phase. However, before the second phase can begin, your pituitary gland has to release two hormones simultaneously, Follicle

Stimulating Hormone (FSH) and Luteinizing Hormone (LH). It is the surge in this hormone that the OPKs detect. This surge is necessary, as it tells the egg follicle that it is time to release and descend through the fallopian tubes and implant itself (if it gets fertilized) into the new lining of your uterus. After this surge is detected, you have a window of about 24 to 36 hours in which your egg can be fertilized. The day after the surge and the day of ovulation are the most fertile days of your cycle. Some people never have a surge detected with OPKs, even though they are, in fact, ovulating. This method requires you to pee on a stick (POAS) during certain days of your cycle. The OPKs will show the surge (or not) through various ways. You can purchase a digital OPK, a simple two-line OPK, or an OPK that shows a happy face or a sad face.

Another way to improve your chances for pregnancy is by charting your cycle. You can find and download charts to write your information on, or try a website like www.fertilityfriend.com to chart the cycle. This method ranges from taking your temperature daily to checking your cervical mucus and cervix position. It starts the first day of your menstrual cycle. You wake up and take your basal body temperature (you will need a basal body thermometer) before you get up, move around, or drink anything. The day before ovulation, your temperature will drop slightly. The day you ovulate it will rise and be higher than your previous temperatures. Once it rises, you've already ovulated. Charting can help you find out when you normally ovulate after a few months of taking your temperature daily. You can also record data on the chart on when you've had sex, what your cervical mucus (CM) looks and feels like, and what your cervical position is. Your cervical mucus changes with the hormones in your body. Before ovulation, your CM goes from sticky and creamy to a watery consistency, and right before ovulation it is an egg white consistency. Don't check your CM after sex, as at that time it can give you false readings. To check it properly, make sure your hands are clean (fingernails too). Sit on a toilet or with one leg on the edge of your tub, insert your fingers as far in as you can and "scoop" out some mucus.

This mucus is the closest to your cervix and, therefore, much purer. The egg white consistency is what you are looking for. This mucus is the one that helps guide the sperm towards its intended target. The cervix position is hard to find if you are not "in tune" with your body. Many women will never find their cervix, and it takes a lot of practice to figure out what it is. Once you find it, feel the texture and record that, as well as position (high, low, or medium). If you can feel the opening, you record that too (open, closed, or medium). Before and during ovulation, your cervix will be high, open, and soft. The softness or hardness of your cervix generally equates to the feel of parts of your face. When it is hard and low, it will feel like the tip of your nose. When it is high and soft, it will feel like your lips. When it is high, it is hard to find. If you've never had a baby, the opening will be small and hard to determine.

For those that don't want to buy OPKs monthly, take their temperature daily, or touch their CM or cervix, there is another way: fertility monitors. Fertility monitors are an easy way to find out when you are about to ovulate. You have to push a button once a day, and then tell you when it's time to POAS. The fertility monitors are expensive, but very helpful. On your first day of menstruation, you start it up. You push the on button when you wake up, and this gives you a six-hour window of time to push that button. This is helpful if your first day of your cycle is on a sleepy Saturday. Once you push the button, it will let count a new day if you push it three hours before or three hours after you first pushed it. During your first cycle, it has your POAS on or around the sixth day of your cycle, and you continue doing this until you ovulate. When you are close to ovulation, it tells you that you are fertile. Again, it's an expensive choice to make, but if you are thinking of having more than one child, it can really help you get pregnant faster.

Having a Baby Is Literally Good for You

Having a baby can make you happier. After you deliver your child, especially if you do it without drugs, your body releases "love" hormones. You feel a sense of euphoria and happiness. You look into your baby's eyes, hold its little hands, and quiver with love for him or her. You'll find yourself smiling more often as you watch the baby grow and thrive. If you breastfeed your infant, you are not only saving money and feeding the baby the only food that is created by your body for the specific needs of your child, but you are also lowering your risk factor for breast cancer.

When to Start Taking Prenatal Vitamins

As soon as you decide to start trying to conceive, start taking your prenatal vitamins. If you have not seen a caregiver, the vitamins can be purchased over-the-counter. Taking them at least two months before conception can help assure that you are getting enough folic acid to reduce the risk of having a baby with neural tube defects like spina bifida. You should look for a prenatal vitamin that has at least 800 mcg of folic acid. The dose for a non-pregnant woman is 400 mcg (.40 mg), and for a pregnant woman it is suggested that you take 800 to 1000 mcg (.80 to 1.0 mg) of folic acid. Some over-the-counter prenatal vitamins contain 800 mcg, but if you want more than that, you usually have to get a prescription.

Chapter 2: Signs of Pregnancy

The Early Signs of Pregnancy

There are many signs of pregnancy and some can be detected as soon as you conceive. The following is a short list of signs which you can use to determine if you are pregnant.

- Missed period

- Spotting during your normal period; shorter and lighter than normal

- Sore breasts

- Fatigue

- Bloating

- Period-like cramps

- Spotting in the middle of your cycle (this could be implantation)

- Nausea

- Strong sense of smell

- Darker areolas or nipples

- Frequent urination

- Food cravings

- Headaches

- Constipation

- Mood swings

While these are signs of pregnancy, a lot of them are also signs of an imminent period. Here are the two ways to determine if you are truly pregnant.

- Take a home pregnancy test (HPT).

Make sure you find one that detects very low levels of Human chorionic gonadotropin (HcG) if you take the test before your period is due.

- Ask your caregiver for a pregnancy blood test.

Especially helpful if you've missed your period, but HPTs are not positive.

Note: if you do not have a positive pregnancy test (either blood test or HPT), you can ask your caregiver for a transvaginal ultrasound. The caregiver may wait a few weeks to be sure you did not have an irregular cycle. It's important that you *act* as though you are pregnant during this time period. Stop smoking, drinking, and taking drugs, and take your prenatal vitamins.

When Do Signs of Pregnancy Typically Start?

These pregnancy signs can start as soon as you conceive, but most often they do not start showing up until you are six weeks along. Some people never have these signs. Recently, a woman I know found out she was pregnant when she was 20-weeks along in her pregnancy. She had unusual cycles, so did not think that there was anything odd about not having her period on a regular basis. She also did not have any of the early pregnancy signs. It wasn't until she felt the baby move that she thought she could be pregnant. This shows that it is wise not to rely on the "typical" signs of pregnancy to show themselves. If you think you may be pregnant, take an HPT.

HPTs range in price from $1.00 to around $15.00. They can be the type of test that you dip into a cup of urine, one you urinate on and these show you lines or plus signs. There are also digital HPTs which shows the words, "Pregnant" and "Not Pregnant." Sometimes, it pays to buy the digital test if you have trouble reading the other tests.

How to Recognize Signs of Pregnancy

If you are in-tune with your body, you may be able to recognize the signs of pregnancy quite early. Some women can feel when they ovulate—a sharp pain on either side of the lower abdomen—a sign that the egg has separated from the ovary and is ready to descend. Some may notice some spotting mid-cycle, which can be a sign that the fertilized egg has been implanted within the uterine walls.

You may notice that sleeping on your tummy hurts your breasts. The breasts can become increasingly sensitive during the first trimester, but usually stop being tender either before or during the second trimester.

Frequent urination and nausea may also be noticed early on. Even though the fetus is only the size of a small seed when you are three to four weeks along, your body is already starting to go through changes. There is a surge of HcG and estrogen. This triggers your body to produce more blood, and all of that excess liquid has to be emptied out. Nausea during pregnancy is common, but the cause is unknown. Many caregivers and researchers think that it may be caused by the surge in estrogen and HcG. Another cause for nausea may be your enhanced sense of smell, which causes you to smell odors you may not have noticed before or to be affected by common smells in a different way than you were when you were not pregnant. Either way, the best way to counter nausea is with ginger: ginger teas, lollipops, sodas, and dietary supplements are all available at local stores. You can try to eat crackers for relief as well. If ginger and crackers are not working for you, or if you are vomiting frequently and unable to keep down any food, talk to your caregiver right away. You may have *Hyperemesis gravidarum*, which is an uncommon pregnancy issue, but can be devastating to your health. *Hyperemesis* is a disorder that can last throughout pregnancy and does not end during the first or second trimester, as normal "morning" sickness does. While morning sickness can happen at any time, morning, noon, and night, *Hyperemesis* occurs throughout the day, whenever you eat or drink. It can cause dehydration, weight-loss, and malnutrition.

Taking a Home Pregnancy Test and HCG Levels

Most home pregnancy tests can now detect pregnancy as early as five days before your period is due. These tests can be both a blessing and a curse. Eggs can be fertilized and implanted, but still be shed with the uterine lining. Many women have "early miscarriages" after they take a sensitive HPT, yet had they not taken the HPT; they would have had their period on-time anyway and never known they'd lost a potential baby. However, peeing on that stick can be supremely addictive. Each time you test, you have the hope of seeing a positive—the dream of a baby. Many chemical pregnancies (HcG and estrogen surge through your body, but there is no actual fetus) are detected early with HPTs.

The sensitive HPTs can detect anywhere from 15mIU(mili International Units, or how much HcG is in each unit of urine) of HcG to 25mIU of HcG. Other tests, usually the cheaper ones and digital tests, only offer a positive when the level of HcG in your system is much higher; some do not register a positive until the level of HcG in your system is 40 to 50mIU. Check the information on the tests at the store (or online) for how much HcG they detect before purchasing one for an early test.

If you are taking a late test, it doesn't really matter what brand you buy, since HcG numbers climb the further along you are in your pregnancy, until around your twelfth week when the levels stop rising. The numbers can go quite high, and usually double every two days, and the numbers differ from woman to woman.

Choosing an OB/GYN or a Midwife

How you decide to birth your baby is up to you, but if you want a natural, medication-free pregnancy, a midwife may be your best choice. Here are some things to expect from both parties.

Obstetrician—

- Hospital delivery

- Medical interventions

Multiple tests, frequent fetal monitoring during labor, ultrasounds for size of baby, pain management

- Little one-on-one time during prenatal appointments, usually about 10 to 15 minutes with the caregiver

- Fetal heartbeat at each appointment (sometimes done by the nurse before the caregiver arrives)

- Ultrasound at 20 weeks

- Not seeing much of the caregiver during labor, until the moment of delivery

- Laboring on your back, delivering on your back (some hospitals allow different positions, some don't)

- Laboring in a tub (but no water births allowed)

- Not allowed to deliver a breech baby naturally (Cesarean only)

- Costly—dependent upon your health insurance. An OB guided pregnancy, without insurance, can cost upwards of $9,000 dollars (not including prenatal care, tests, or ultrasounds), and you will receive a separate bill for baby.

Midwife—

- Hospital delivery (in some areas, they cannot offer a hospital birth by law), birthing center delivery, and home birth delivery.

- Few medical interventions

Tests taken how you want, when necessary, fetal monitoring during labor is done with a stethoscope, no pain management—natural, drug-free births only

- A lot of one-on-one time during appointments, usually about 30 to 60 minutes, depending on how much you want to talk about

- Fetal heartbeat at each appointment

- Ultrasound at 20 weeks (and no more unless medical problems arise)

- Nearly constant presence during labor and delivery

- Laboring however you want, delivering in the position/way most comfortable for you

- Water birth

- Will attempt to deliver most breech positions

- Cost of delivery/prenatal care is usually below $3500 out of pocket (but you may be charged extra for tests and ultrasounds)

The difference arises because OBs are trained to treat pregnancy the same way they treat diseases, while midwives are trained to treat pregnancy as a natural part of life. This doesn't make OBs a bad choice in any way; it all depends on your level of comfort. Some women want the OBs around; want the hospital experience, fearful of anything that could possibly go wrong. Some women find this choice to be too constricting and know that the midwife will not let them deliver at home or at the birthing center if a problem arises. If you are having a difficult labor, decide you want an epidural, or if the baby is showing distress, the midwife will call an ambulance and have you taken to the hospital. Most caregivers will not allow you to deliver a baby that is breech, because they have not been trained to deliver breech babies. Midwives undergo hours and hours of training, some of their training is in developing countries, and they are trained to deliver most breech positions.

To find a provider, make multiple consultation appointments with the candidates you've chosen. Have a list of questions ready. Some questions to ask are

- What is your C-section rate? (If they are higher than ten percent, it could be a red flag for you.);

- How long will I be allowed to remain pregnant before induction? (The estimated due date is just that, an estimation. First time pregnancies can go on for 38 – 42 weeks, and some delivery naturally at 43 weeks.)

- Will you be available (not on vacation) around the time of my due date?

- Will you make every effort to follow my birth plan?

- At which hospitals are you allowed to deliver?

- How long are your prenatal appointments?

- When are certain tests due, and can I opt-out of taking any?

You may be able to think of further questions to ask each OB or midwife. One thing to watch for is the attention the OB or midwife gives to you while you are consulting with them. Pay close attention to the details. Are they fidgety? Do they train all of their attention on you, or do they look like they are in a hurry? Do you feel comfortable in their presence? If you aren't comfortable around someone fully-clothed, you won't be comfortable barely-clothed and exposed.

The First Prenatal Appointment: What to Expect

Your first prenatal appointment can be scheduled anywhere from seven weeks to nine weeks, depending on your past history and how busy your caregiver is. As soon as your pregnancy is detected, call the caregiver or midwife to make an appointment.

The first appointment is generally longer than any of the other appointments, except for the appointment in which the caregiver or midwife tests for Gestational Diabetes. The caregiver or midwife will determine your due date based on your last menstrual cycle or from when you ovulated. You will be asked if you've had past pregnancies, and if you have, what was the result? They will want to know about past surgeries. You will be asked for your medical history, including that of your father and mother. They will want to know if you smoke, drink, or take drugs (and how often) and what, if any, prescription or over-the-counter medications you are currently taking. Here are some tests that may be performed.

- A urine test to check for bladder infection, kidney disease, and sugars (they may also use it for an additional pregnancy test);

- a blood test (a complete blood count (CBC) which checks for blood problems;

- an HIV test (which is optional, but if you've never had one, take it);

- a test for Rubella (they are looking for immunity);

- a test for immunity to Chicken Pox;

- a hepatitis B test;

- a blood type test to determine if you are Rh+ or Rh- (if this is a first-time pregnancy, the father should be tested as well);

- you can ask for genetic testing, in which both you and your spouse will be tested for genetic markers for certain diseases;

- a pelvic exam (your caregiver will perform a pap smear if one is due, but not if you've had one within the last two years. He or she will also insert two fingers until they touch your cervix, and then he or she will press down on your uterus to try and determine how big your uterus is).

Placenta: How It Works

The placenta is a marvelous invention in evolution. It eliminates wastes, helps feed the baby nutrients, and exchanges gasses via the mother's blood. It starts to form as soon as the blastocyst (the egg, while it is still splitting into many cells) implants in the uterine lining. As your baby grows, the placenta grows. The blood flow from mama to baby is fully developed in the placenta by the beginning of the second trimester. The umbilical cord goes from placenta to baby, and it is much like a two-way street. Wastes from the baby are returned through the umbilical cord to the placenta, while fresh nutrients are delivered. A healthy placenta is a working placenta that will help your baby grow and thrive.

Danger Signs in Early Pregnancy

Early pregnancy is both exhilarating and highly emotional. It is when you truly form the over-protective worrier part of your psyche. It is when you first discover how scary bringing a new life into this world can be, and that fear of something horrible happening to your child never leaves you. Some problems that can occur in early pregnancy can be avoided if you seek medical attention right away, but sadly, some cannot. Call your caregiver

- if you start cramping badly. Never think that anything is too inconsequential—it could mean the difference between life and death;

- if you notice fresh blood (it will be bright red, not brown, which is old blood, and it can contain clots, be abundant or sparse);

- if you develop a fever or get the chills (this could be a sign of an infection and an elevated temperature can damage the fetus);

- if you feel faint;

- if you have frequent, painful urination (this could be a bladder infection);

- if you have a fever and are also vomiting.

If any of these symptoms appear, it is imperative that you see your caregiver as soon as possible. If your caregiver is not available or if it is nighttime, call the help line they provide and/or go to the emergency room. If the problem is an infection, a cold, or placenta previa, the caregiver will be able to help control the problem; however, if it is placenta previa, then your midwife will not be able to help you as you will require a C-section. Don't feel like you are calling your caregiver too often, especially if you feel something is just not right. At the least, they can give you a peace of mind, at the most, they can help divert disaster or prepare you for it.

Chapter 3: Vitamins and Supplements

Choosing Your Pregnancy Supplements

The prenatal vitamin is a mix of many different nutrients that are needed for a healthy pregnancy. Choosing one can be difficult, as some can irritate your stomach, cause nausea if you are already pregnant, and may not contain the amount of nutrients you need to maintain a healthy pregnancy. Work with your caregiver to find the right supplement for you. If the prenatal vitamins you try cause too many issues, they can help you find a mixture that will work well.

How Does Folic Acid Support a Healthy Pregnancy?

Folic acid is a staple in prenatal vitamins. However, it can also be found in certain foods. A diet rich in folate (folic acid) can reduce the risks of birth defects that affect the brain, such as spina bifida. Some foods that contain folate are

- Asparagus

- Spinach

- Avocado

- Peanuts

- Romaine lettuce

- Orange juice

These are just a few of the foods; there are many foods out there that contain folate. If you take your vitamins in conjunction with eating well, you are paving the way towards a healthy pregnancy.

Why Is Iron Important?

Iron helps your blood move through your body, forms hemoglobin, supports your immune system, and helps your baby's brain develop.

Starting from the moment of conception, your blood volume starts increasing. Your blood volume will increase to about 45% of its normal capacity. Anemia is common in pregnant women who do not get enough iron, which not only affects the woman, but also the fetus. The baby stores up iron in its system, which lasts until they are three to six months old.

There are many foods that contain iron and will help keep your iron levels up. Some are

- Clams

- White beans

- Kidney beans

- Red meat

- Pumpkin seeds

These are only a few; more can be found through research, or by asking your caregiver.

Benefits of Fish Oil during Pregnancy

Some prenatal vitamins have DHA (a form of fish oil) added to them. DHA is thought to support fetal brain and eye development, and some studies have shown that getting 200 mg of DHA daily can increase your gestational period by at least four days. It is believed to reduce the risks of

- Postpartum depression

- Cerebral palsy

- Gestational diabetes

- Preeclampsia

- Premature birth

Although it helps prevent these risks, it does not necessarily mean they will disappear. Taking DHA supplements can make it less likely that you'll develop these problems during your pregnancy, but other factors may increase your risks, and sometimes, things just happen no matter what you do.

The Amount of Vitamins Needed for a Healthy Pregnancy

Remember that prenatal vitamins are just supplements, and you should also consume foods that are rich in these nutrients. Because they are just supplements, you may read the ingredients on the back of the prenatal vitamins and find, "Vitamin A 4,000 IU" and in the column marked % of daily value, "50%." This means the other 50% should be in foods you consume.

If your caregiver does not prescribe prenatal vitamins and tells you that you can use over-the-counter vitamins, read the back of the bottles and look for pills with these minimum amounts of nutrients

- Vitamin A—4,000 IU (international units)

- Folic Acid—800 – 1,000 mcg

- Vitamin D—200-400 IU

- Calcium—200-300 milligrams (mg)

- Vitamin C—85+ mcg

- Thiamin—1.4+ mg

- Riboflavin—1.4+ mg

- Vitamin B-6—2.6 mg

- Niacin (or B3)—18 mg

- Vitamin B12—4 mcg

- Vitamin E—15 mcg or 11 IU

- Zinc—11+ mg

- Iron—27-60 mg

If the pills do not have these minimums, either buy additional supplements or find a brand that does.

Chapter 4: Tests That Can Be Performed during Pregnancy

Types of Tests That Are Routinely Done at the Doctor's Office

In addition to the tests you will receive at your first office visit, there are other tests that your caregiver may perform throughout your pregnancy.

One test you will be asked to take is the AFP testing, sometimes called triple screen or quad screen. It tests for neural tube defects like spina bifida. Sometimes, it is used to detect Downs Syndrome. This test is generally performed between 15 and 17 weeks of pregnancy. It is a simple blood test, either drawn at the caregiver's office, or at a lab or hospital. The test is most sensitive in the time period stated, and if your dates are off by a little bit, the results can be false. If the test turns out positive, you will have to do further, more invasive testing. The positive results lead to a level two ultrasound or an amniocentesis. Because of the large amount of false positives, and depending on your belief system, you can decline this test and wait for the 20 week ultrasound. If you would keep the pregnancy going regardless of the outcome, then this test is unnecessary, and you can decline it.

Another early test is the Nuchal Translucency screening, in which they test for Downs Syndrome. This test is done between weeks 11 to 14 of your pregnancy, and is done with an ultrasound. The ultrasound can detect the thickness of the nuchal fold. If it is thick, your risk is higher. If it comes back positive, they may ask you to get an amniocentesis or a chorionic villus sampling (CVS).

The amniocentesis can be used to find out if your baby has a chromosomal disorder in early pregnancy. If done during the third trimester, it is looking for your baby's lung maturity (only if you are to be induced or go into premature labor after 34 weeks). It is accomplished by the doctor placing a small needle through the abdomen into the uterus. They also perform an ultrasound at the same time, to help guide the needle away from baby or placenta. They take a sample of the amniotic fluid which they test for chromosomal disorders. This test can be performed as early as 11 weeks.

The CVS test is much like the amniocentesis, but can be performed at 8 weeks. The doctor uses a needle and an ultrasound, but instead of only going in through the abdomen, the doctor can also go in through the vagina near the uterus. The CVS test gathers a small sample of villi to look for genetic disorders. The results show either a normal baby or a genetic defect and can also identify gender. Both the amniocentesis and the CVS test have a risk for miscarriage, though it is very low, from about 1-2%.

Other tests that are done during pregnancy are

- Gestational Diabetes tests –usually around 24 – 28 weeks

- Ultrasounds

- Non-stress test (NST)—usually approaching your due date or if you have any problems during pregnancy. This checks to see if baby is stressed or not, usually done if you are past your due date.

- Biophysical profile (BPP)—also done towards due date or if any problems are present. This test checks for muscle tone, breathing movements, and the level of amniotic fluid, usually done if you are past your due date.

- Group B Streptococcus (GBS)—this is done to see if you have GBS around your vagina. It's a simple swab test that is usually done towards your due date. If you are positive, the baby can contract it on the way out, so at the hospital, they will give you intravenous antibiotics every two hours, at least twice. The midwife may have other options.

Ultrasounds: Why Do Them and What Are They Used for?

Ultrasounds can be used to guide needles for the CVS and amniocentesis, to perform the BPP, and to help date (if you are unsure of when you conceived) and track the baby's growth. The 20 week ultrasound is when most women find out the sex of their baby, but contrary to popular belief, that's not why it's done. They measure the baby's heart and make sure it is growing correctly, measure the head, the bones, the kidneys and the stomach. They look at the umbilical cord and watch the blood flow to affirm that is operating properly. They measure the heartbeat. The technician performing the ultrasound cannot give you the results. The results are sent to your caregiver, and they translate the results for you.

When Should I Decline Testing?

You should decline testing if you find it unnecessary or if you find it medically invasive. Some testing shouldn't be declined, like the GBS test or the gestational diabetes test. You can decline most tests; however, if you do, your caregiver may have you sign an "against medical advice" (AMA) form for their own safety.

Chapter 5: Pregnancy Diet

A Healthy Diet Is Important during Pregnancy

A healthy diet is important during pregnancy because it helps your baby grow and keeps you healthy as well. If you are not getting enough nutrients for yourself, your baby still gets them. The baby strips your body of the nutrients it needs to grow. Therefore, if you are not getting the minimum amount of nutrients needed, you are the one who goes without. So if you are the type of person that eats takeout on a daily basis, a switch in diet is needed if you are thinking of becoming pregnant or if you are already pregnant.

What Are Some Healthy Pregnancy Diets?

There are a lot of healthy pregnancy diets to be found on the internet or in pregnancy books, so I am not going to outline every single one. However, here are *some* foods to start integrating into your diet if you are pregnant or thinking of becoming pregnant.

- Legumes: *Contains protein, iron and folic acid*

- Meat (poultry, lean meat, fish): *Contains protein and iron*

- Dairy (milk, yogurt, cheese, pudding): *Contains calcium, protein, vitamin B, and vitamin D*

- Fresh Fruit: *Contains vitamin C*

- Vegetables (sweet corn, broccoli, asparagus, yeast extract): *Contains folic acid and iron*

Remember the old FDA food pyramid? It was like a one size fits all dress that neglected half of the population, because it wasn't really made for everyone. The new FDA food guidelines from www.choosemyplate.gov give you the ability to choose what's right for you. The guidelines are based on the FDA's 2005 Dietary guidelines and provide an image of a plate that shows you how much of each food should be on your plate.

If you go to the website provided, you can enter your information into their form and it will provide an individualized meal plan made just for you. For instance, if you are a 120 pound, 28-year old woman, with less than 30 minutes of exercise per day, it tells you to eat

- 6 ounces of grains

- 2.5 cups of vegetables

- 1.5 cups of fruit

- 4 cups of dairy

- 5 ounces of protein.

These are the daily amounts you should eat if that is your physical make-up. It includes helpful tips near each food group, explaining what foods to look for in that category. You can create a profile and track your diet, as well as your exercise, on the website. This is a wonderful resource for everyone. You can start using it before you conceive and learn how to eat right beforehand.

Choosing Healthy Snacks

A great way to choose a healthy snack is to follow the Food Guide Plate at www.choosemyplate.gov/food-groups. This page shows how much the foods count towards your daily allowance. For instance, if you click on fruit, and then apple, it will pop-up a picture of an apple, and then it will tell you how many cups of fruit it contains.

Choose snacks that are nutritious and avoid snacks that are packed with fat and sugars. Your snacks should be part of your healthy, balanced diet. When you start following your healthy diet, make lists before you go to the store. One way to avoid buying sugary, fatty snacks is to eat before you head off to the grocery store. You'll find that you buy less off-the-list items, and it will be easier to stick to your list.

Foods to Avoid while Pregnant

A lot of women don't realize that there are foods you just should not eat while pregnant. It can get very hard to avoid the foods, because you may find yourself craving them, but remembering that you are staying healthy for your baby, as well as for yourself, can make it a bit easier to handle. If there is a food on this list that you crave throughout pregnancy, have your significant other buy it when you are in labor, or after you have given birth. It can be your celebratory feast! Here are the foods to avoid:

Cold deli meats—deli meats can contain listeria, which can cause miscarriages. It can cross into the placenta and could infect the baby. If you just *have* to have deli meat, reheat it until it is steaming, not warm.

Raw Meat—raw meats can contain all sorts of contaminations, and while pregnant, should be avoided.

Fish containing mercury—some fish are contaminated with mercury. There are levels of mercury in fish, some contain high mercury levels, and some contain low mercury levels. Your caregiver can give you information on how much to eat a week, but the FDA says you can eat at least 12 ounces of low mercury fish weekly. A few fish to avoid (not the extensive list) are shark, Ahi tuna, and marlin. You can eat six ounces of sea bass, canned tuna, and yellow tuna a month. You can have 12 ounces of perch, crawfish, catfish, clams, shrimp, tilapia, and salmon a week. The latter list is quite extensive, so don't feel like you are limited too much if you love fish.

- Raw and smoked seafood—these contain a plethora of contaminates that can affect you during pregnancy and should be avoided altogether. This means no raw oysters or any type of sushi—even sushi made with cooked fish has a chance to be contaminated. They usually make the cooked sushi on the same surfaces.

- Raw eggs—since there is a danger of salmonella contamination with eggs, it's best to avoid any foods that contain raw eggs, such as: Caesar salad dressings, mayonnaise, homemade custards, or undercooked eggs.

- Soft cheeses—these are mostly imported and can contain listeria. These include Brie, Roquefort, Feta, and Mexican *quesoblanco* cheeses.

Always remember to wash your vegetables, especially if you do your own gardening. The soil can contain toxoplasmosis, thanks to the neighborhood cats, and can potentially cause a rare blood infection.

Healthy Pregnancy Eating Habits

Don't let the old saying, "I'm eating for two now, I can eat what I want," take over your life while pregnant. This can lead to overeating, eating a lot of junk food, and gaining too much weight. Don't think of this new eating regimen as a diet, either. This is a lifestyle change, and there isn't anything that says you can't continue eating that way once you have the baby. Pregnant women need about 2200-2500 calories daily, which is more than the normal amount for non-pregnant women. It isn't a huge difference though, and that is where some women make the mistake of overeating. A normal, healthy woman consumes around 1600-2200 calories a day. Check the back of products for food serving sizes and calories per serving. Also look at how much sodium and fat each serving contains. If you find the results to be higher than expected, it's because it is overly processed; try cooking fresh ingredients to make the same product. Pencil in a little bit of extra time into your day to cook your meals, and you'll love the results.

How to Control Pregnancy Junk Food Cravings

Controlling junk food cravings can be difficult. Don't take this food out of your diet completely, or you may end up binging and eating far too much. Instead, buy small amounts (1 serving size) for that moment when you most definitely cannot substitute something else. There are substitutions that may mull you over until the next craving hits. For instance, instead of eating potato chips, try some pretzels or low-fat popcorn. You can substitute a low-fat granola bar for a candy bar or raisins and dried fruits for crunchy candies. Trail mix (without chocolate) can be a great substitute as well. Instead of ice cream, try yogurt or pudding. If you want a soda, drink fruit juice. If it is the bubbles you crave, you can buy seltzer water to put in your fruit juice. Do what you can to avoid junk food, but don't beat yourself up if you give in every now and then.

How Much Water Do You Need?

Drinking water helps keep you hydrated. It also helps carry nutrients through your body. The rule of thumb is to drink *at least* eight 8-ounce glasses of fluid per day; however, it doesn't necessarily have to be plain water. You can drink juices, milk, and drinks that contain caffeine or are decaffeinated. You should, however, limit your intake of caffeine. Drink when thirsty and during light activity. Dehydration can trigger early labor; if you start contracting early (and it isn't painful) drink water and lie down. If your legs and ankles or hands swell, drink more water. Drinking water is not what makes you retain water, and drinking more can actually help reduce the swelling.

Chapter 6: Fitness in Pregnancy

How Does Fitness Help You Have a Healthy Pregnancy?

Getting fit, or staying fit, during pregnancy can help combat high blood pressure, aches and pains, and reduce your risk of getting gestational diabetes or having a C-section.

Tips for Healthy Exercise during Pregnancy

If you are exercising before pregnancy, continue exercising normally, usually until you find it uncomfortable or on the advice of your caregiver. Remain hydrated while exercising. If you experience pain or cramping while exercising, stop. Always ask your caregiver which exercises are safe and which are not. If you are not currently exercising or are sedentary, you can start by walking daily. You can safely walk from 30 – 60 minutes a day, and it doesn't all have to be at one time, nor does it need to be a power walk.

How Pregnancy Yoga Helps You Keep Fit and Healthy

Yoga not only helps you stay fit during pregnancy, but it can also help you deliver your baby. Yoga helps your body be flexible, and enables you to use a variety of positions during labor. It makes helps you remain calm and reduces stress. In can improve your posture, which can help with back problems associated with pregnancy. It can strengthen your pelvic floor, and after pregnancy, it can strengthen your abdominal muscles, which have been stretched out by pregnancy.

What is a Healthy Pregnancy Weight Gain?

A healthy pregnancy weight gain varies from woman to woman. The average weight gain is 30 pounds, but can greatly vary. Your caregiver will keep track of your weight and make sure you are within acceptable limits. If you are obese, you may even lose weight and the caregiver won't bat an eye, unless it is because you are not getting enough to eat.

Typically, you should gain 1 to 4 pounds during the entire first trimester. After that, you can gain 2 to 4 pounds each month in the next two trimesters. You may find that you gain more towards the end.

How to Not Gain Too Much Weight during Pregnancy

To keep from gaining too much weight, follow a healthy diet and exercise regularly. If you are on bed rest you won't be able to exercise, but you can still eat well. Avoid gorging yourself on chips, candy, and soda pop. Remember that dessert doesn't need to follow every dinner.

Chapter 7: Sex during Pregnancy

How to Have Sex during Pregnancy

You can have sex anyway you like during pregnancy, especially if you have an uncomplicated, low-risk pregnancy; most of the time the only thing that stops you from doing a certain position is your own personal comfort. You can even continue to use sex toys during pregnancy— just don't penetrate too deeply and keep them clean to avoid infections. Oral sex isn't off the table either, but towards the end your significant other may not feel comfortable down there with all the extra fluids your body is producing. Remember that sex doesn't hurt the baby at all. If sex is not safe for you, your caregiver will let you know.

Some of the best sexual positions for pregnancy are side-to-side, missionary, woman-on-top, and intercourse from behind. The further along you are in your pregnancy, the less comfortable some positions may become. Feel free to experiment and let your significant other know if you are uncomfortable or in pain. If you are not comfortable having sex, keep being intimate with your partner. You can mutually masturbate, touch, fondle, and kiss each other. Don't let your discomfort get in the way of your relationship. You may just find that the occasional non-traditional sexual contact actually strengthens your relationship.

What Are the Benefits of Sex during Pregnancy?

There are many benefits that having sex with your partner can have for you, as long as you are in a monogamous relationship, and there is no fear of contracting sexually transmitted diseases. Some of the benefits are that it

- relaxes the baby—the rocking motion and the gentle squeezing of the uterus as your orgasm rocks the baby to sleep;

- induces labor if your body is already geared towards labor—although this is unsubstantiated by any scientific studies, many caregivers still suggest it;

- helps you bond with your significant other—sex can help you become closer to your significant other during an often stressful time in your relationship;

- prepares the pelvic floor for labor—sex helps tones the muscles you will be using when it's time for baby to arrive;

- feels wonderful—your body is changing, and with those changes you will find new and wonderful sensations that you'd probably not felt before.

Oral sex can also help stimulate labor. Recent studies have shown that the prostaglandins found in semen actually help start labor better if the semen is swallowed. This isn't for everyone, though!

When is Sex Allowed and When Is It Not Allowed?

There are multiple reasons why you may be told not to have sex. Most of the reasons revolve around pregnancy complications. Sex will more than likely be outlawed by your caregiver if

- You have gone into preterm labor,

- You have placenta previa,

- Your water breaks,

- You have a history of miscarriages,

- You have an incompetent cervix,

- You experience heavy bleeding.

Remember if your doctor says you cannot have sex, it means no orgasms either.

Chapter 8: Healthy Sleeping in Pregnancy

Sleep during Pregnancy

Getting to sleep while pregnant, especially towards the end of the pregnancy, can be difficult, however, it is not impossible. During your first trimester you won't have any trouble, and will generally sleep more often.

What Sleeping Positions Are Good during Pregnancy?

Sleeping on your left side is the best position for sleeping during pregnancy, especially towards your third trimester. You may find it more comfortable to prop yourself up with pillows if you are experiencing heartburn. Avoid sleeping on your back, as this places pressure on the aorta and the vena cava, which can decrease the circulation to your body and to your baby. It can also increase the chances of heartburn, hemorrhoids, and low blood pressure.

Sleeping Better throughout the Pregnancy

Here are a few tips on how to get better sleep throughout pregnancy.

- Stop drinking caffeinated drinks, which should be limited anyway. If you must drink them, avoid doing so before bedtime.

- Do not drink fluids before bedtime or eat a full meal before sleep.

- Create a routine for waking up and going to sleep at the same time each night.

- Take a warm bath (not too hot) before bed and relax.

- Get up and read or listen to music, something to take your mind off of the fact that you can't sleep if you are tossing and turning and getting angry.

- Buy a body pillow to help alleviate aches throughout the night. There are also special "pregnancy" pillows that you can buy that are created to fit a pregnant body.

Chapter 9: Oral Care during Pregnancy

How to Care for Your Teeth during Pregnancy

Brush your teeth as normal during pregnancy and floss regularly. When you are growing a baby, you need extra calcium, and if you aren't getting enough calcium, your body takes it from your teeth and bones. See your dentist during your first trimester for a cleaning if you haven't already and get any cavities taken care of as soon as possible.

Why Are Your Gums Sensitive During Pregnancy?

During pregnancy, your body is undergoing many changes due to hormones. The higher than normal progesterone levels and the higher blood level can make your gums more sensitive during pregnancy. When your gums swell, they hold in cavity-causing bacteria, which in turn irritates the gums and make them swell even more. Many pregnant women get cavities near their gum line for this reason.

Bleeding Gums during Pregnancy

Since your gums are more sensitive, you will notice some pink in the sink when you brush and floss your teeth. This is due to the pregnancy hormones and your high blood level. This is a normal pregnancy complaint, known as pregnancy gingivitis. The reason you are experiencing more bleeding in your gums than normal, as I stated, is because the hormonal changes make your gums much more sensitive to the bacteria that cause plaque and gingivitis. Don't worry, it doesn't mean you are at a higher risk of having gingivitis after the pregnancy is over. Just go to the dentist regularly to get your teeth cleaned, and brush and floss at least twice a day.

How Cavities Can Affect Your Pregnancy

Even women who don't normally get cavities may find they suddenly get more while pregnant. When your gums swell, they trap food and bacteria, which not only causes bleeding, but also creates cavities at the gum line. The best time to get dental work done is during your second trimester. During the first trimester, your fetus is developing organs, and it is at its most vulnerable, since it is not relying entirely upon the placenta until the second trimester. Because of this, it is best to avoid introducing your fetus to unwanted chemicals and x-rays. Lying on your back for extended periods of time can be hard on your back during the third trimester. Naturally, it's best to wait until after the delivery to get your cavities fixed, but if there is an emergency, Novocain and some antibiotics are safe to use during pregnancy. Most dentists will not order a full set of x-rays when you are pregnant, but if the tooth is bad enough, they may x-ray that one tooth.

But can cavities and gum issues affect the fetus? The simple answer is yes, they can. Uncontrolled gum disease can cause premature birth and low birth weight. Further, women who have cavities while pregnant have children who are more likely to have cavities before the age of five. If you have a cavity that is inflamed or abscessed, it is slowly delivering the poison from the infection into your blood stream, and your blood stream is what is feeding the baby. Get any bad cavities fixed before you become pregnant, or as soon as possible after conception.

Chapter 10: Work Meets Pregnancy

Working during Pregnancy: Do's and Don'ts

There is no reason why a woman can't continue working if they become pregnant. Unless you are told to stop working by your caregiver, you can continue working up until you go into labor.

- Do stay away from smells that can trigger nausea or vomiting.

- Do snack often—keep crackers or Melba toast with you to help alleviate nausea.

- Do keep ginger ale or tea handy.

- Do drink fluids—have bottles of water or a personal water cup filled and with you at all times.

- Don't work until you drop.

- Do take breaks.

- Do walk around—stand up and walk around if you sit often, sit down and relax if your position calls for a lot of standing.

- Don't hide your pregnancy from your boss. It's important that they know you are pregnant and may need extra breaks. Otherwise, they may think you are not doing your job!

What Can You Do to Promote a Healthy Pregnancy at Work?

If your work carries risk, mention them to your caregiver. You may need to modify your work if what you do can be harmful to a growing baby. Some work can cause complications during pregnancy, especially if you are at risk for preterm labor. For instance, if you work around harmful chemicals, large machines, extreme cold environments, or excessive noise, you should find out if you can be moved to a safer position until after delivery. After you have spoken to your caregiver, speak to your boss about the possible problems.

Be sure to relax often and don't overdo it. If you find yourself becoming too stressed out, take a break and breathe. Find a dark place to sit until you are calmer. Talk to the person(s) who are causing stress, or with a friend or coworker. Talking out your problems can help alleviate the stress behind them.

How Does the Stress Level at Your Job Affect a Healthy Pregnancy?

Any type of stress can affect pregnancy, but job-related stress is usually at the top of the charts. Stress sends chemical (cortisol) signals through your body and into your placenta. Cortisol can cross the placenta; however, the exposure of cortisol to a fetus over long periods has not been completely studied. Long term levels of cortisol exposure in adults can lead to depression, exhaustion, and high blood pressure. This could affect your pregnancy by making it harder to work, harder to care about anything, and high blood pressure could lead to preeclampsia. Remember that you are not only growing and caring for a baby, but you also need to start caring for your own health. You can lower your work-related stress by

- Exercising regularly

- Taking a prenatal yoga class

- Learning relaxation techniques for pregnancy

- Relaxing and taking a breather when the stress levels get too high

- Walking

- Breathing deeply (breathe in slowly through your nose to the count of five, exhale slowly through your mouth for the count of eight. Repeat.)

- Cuddling with your spouse or pet

- Getting a pregnancy massage

- Listening to relaxing music

- Thinking positively

You can control the amount of stress you are feeling at work and at home. The hardest part is letting go of the stress your work is causing instead of stewing over it angrily.

Chapter 11: Common Pregnancy Ailments

Yeast Infection during Pregnancy

Yeast lives in warm, wet, sweet, dark places. It thrives most during pregnancy, because of the extra wetness pregnancy hormones create, and the increase of sugar in your discharge. You may notice you have more discharge while you are pregnant. If that discharge has an odd smell to it, sometimes accompanied by itchiness, it may be a yeast infection. Don't rely on self-diagnosis though, instead, mention it to your caregiver. It is a fast, easy test and it could be a different vaginal infection, like Bacterial Vaginosis, which can cause premature birth. The antibiotic Diflucan, which is usually prescribed to non-pregnant women, has not been proven safe for pregnancy. Instead, your caregiver will give you a prescription or recommend an antibacterial suppository or cream, which you will apply for 7 – 14 days.

Pregnancy Constipation: Are Stool Softeners Safe?

Constipation is a common side effect of pregnancy. There are a few over-the-counter stool softeners that are safe to take during pregnancy (don't take laxatives during pregnancy); however, speak to your caregiver to find out what is best for you. If you want to avoid using medications, there are natural alternatives to stool softeners.

- Drink more water

- Drink prune juice

- Eat foods with high fiber

- Eat raisins, apples, bananas and rhubarb

How to Have a Healthy Pregnancy with Hypertension

You can have normal blood pressure when you aren't pregnant, and then suddenly your caregiver finds your blood pressure to be a bit higher than normal. Blood pressure is usually considered high once it reaches 140/90+. A normal reading is usually around 130/70. If you are getting high blood pressure readings your caregiver will start to pay very close attention to it. High blood pressure during pregnancy can cause

- Premature delivery—if your blood pressure is too high, your caregiver may opt for a premature delivery to prevent any life-threatening conditions for you or for the baby.

- Decreased blood flow to the placenta—placenta is the life force for your baby. A decreased blood flow means that the baby isn't getting enough oxygen or nutrients, which can lead to IUGR (inter uterine growth retardation) or SGA (small for gestational age) which in turn could lead to premature delivery.

- Placental abruption—this can cause problems for both the baby and the mother and is considered a life-threatening condition for the baby, as they are deprived of nutrients and oxygen. It could lead to a C-section.

- Preeclampsia—this disorder usually manifests towards the end of pregnancy, but can also manifest earlier or even after delivery. Preeclampsia is life-threatening and can result in early induction or a C-section.

If you are already hypertensive and are on medication prior to pregnancy, speak to your caregiver about your medications and make sure they are safe to take while pregnant. If you are diagnosed with high blood pressure during pregnancy, your caregiver may prescribe medication to treat it. Some blood pressure medications are considered safe for pregnancy, and while most medications do cross the placenta and contain risks to the baby, your caregiver will decide on whether to prescribe the medications on risk versus the reward. If the risk of the medication outweighs the reward, they won't prescribe it.

You can lower your blood pressure by exercising and eating healthy. Look at diets that call for natural ingredients. Watch documentaries such as *Forks over Knives* to learn how eating right can increase your own health and decrease your reliance on medications.

How to Prevent Stretch Marks during Pregnancy

When your body grows quickly, your skin stretches to keep up with your body's growth. During pregnancy, it grows very quickly. One day you wake up and suddenly you *look* pregnant. When your skin is stretching rapidly, the elastin can be damaged and create stretch marks. There are a lot of creams and ointments on the market that claim to prevent stretch marks, but the truth of the matter is that you can't prevent stretch marks. Stretch marks have more to do with your genetic make-up than with what creams or ointments you slather on your belly. If your mother made it through pregnancy without stretch marks, chances are you won't have any either—or very few. While ointments and creams won't prevent stretch marks, however, they can lessen the appearance of stretch marks, and that's when these products come in handy. Look for natural creams and ointments, though, as a lot of commercial products contain ingredients that can be harmful and have not been tested for safety of use during pregnancy. Also, if you have sensitive skin, they can wreak havoc on you and give you sleepless nights. The best way to prevent or soften the look of stretch marks is to decrease stress, increase fluids, keep skin hydrated with natural oils or creams (try vitamin E), eat nutritional foods, and watch your weight gain. Most importantly, if you do get stretch marks, don't let them upset you. They are a mark of motherhood and only truly beautiful women wear them proudly. Also, they tend to stop being red and angry as the years go by, and turn into soft, silvery lines that can only be seen in certain lights.

What Helps to Relieve Swollen Feet during Pregnancy?

There are a few ways to reduce and relieve swollen feet during pregnancy. Here are a few things you can try.

- Drink more water! While fluid retention is one of the causes of swollen feet, drinking more water can actually help relieve that swelling. Water retention generally occurs as a way for your body to retain water when you are not getting enough.

- Put your feet up.

- Stay off your feet for long hours at a time.

- Wear shoes that fit properly. Now is the time to get rid of the high heels. Also, your feet change size during pregnancy, be sure you are measuring them throughout pregnancy.

- Give your feet a water bath in Epsom salts.

- Ask your partner to give you a foot massage to help soothe the discomfort.

Tips on How to Relieve Pelvic Pressure during the Last Trimester

As you approach your due date, you may notice extra pressure in your pelvic floor. Sometimes, it feels like the baby's head is *right there*, ready to come out, and it isn't a comfortable feeling. As you progress in your pregnancy, the baby starts to position itself to prepare for birth. This position can be uncomfortable and there are a few things you can try to relieve that comfort, though the only real way to rid yourself of it entirely is to give birth.

- Lay on your left side

- Use a belly band or sling, it helps support your uterus

- Change positions

- Take a warm bath

- Position yourself on your hands and knees and rest your head between your hands leaving your butt up in the air for 20 minute intervals.

This last position can help relieve the pressure, as well as position baby better, open the pelvic floor, and relieve back pain.

Chapter 12: Complications That Can Occur

What is Gestational Diabetes?

Even if you've never had diabetes before, eat healthy, and are not overweight, you can be diagnosed as having gestational diabetes. There is no hard evidence on *why* it happens, but in some pregnancies, the body just isn't able to produce enough insulin to control the blood sugar. When you're pregnant and your blood sugars are elevated above normal, you will be asked to take your blood sugar four times a day and, in some cases, record your daily food intake. If you are unable to keep your levels down by diet alone, you may be prescribed insulin. The reason they watch closely for gestational diabetes is that it can have negative effects on the baby.

Gestational diabetes can give your baby high blood glucose levels, which makes the baby's pancreas increase insulin levels, it gets more energy and turns that energy into fat, leading to macrosomia (a fat baby). Macrosomia can

Lead to future weight problems

Increase the child's risk for adult onset type 2 diabetes

Cause shoulder dystocia during birth

Cause breathing problems in newborns

Cause low blood sugar at birth

The blood glucose test is typically run during the 24th to the 28th week depending on your doctor. It generally affects the mother after the baby's body has finished forming (it has all its digits and looks like a baby) but before they've completely grown in size or weight. The best way to avoid gestational diabetes or to control it once you've been diagnosed is to eat a healthy diet low in sugars and processed foods.

What is Fetal Demise?

Fetal demise is the medical terminology for a baby that has died in the womb. Even healthy pregnancies can suddenly turn for the worst. The baby that was once moving and playing inside your tummy suddenly stops, and sometimes, there is no discernible reason or cause for the baby's demise. If it happens to you, the best thing to do is to talk about your feelings with your partner, join other mothers who have experienced a loss, or even join a support group for women who have experienced a loss. Give yourself time to grieve. Losing a baby at any stage of pregnancy is devastating to both of you. Your partner may not seem like he is hurting the same way you are, but he is. Everyone grieves in their own way, it is important that they are given the time to do so.

There is nothing that can prepare you for it, even when you know you are giving birth to a stillborn, you hold out hope that maybe all the doctors were wrong and your baby will cry. You will feel its heartbeat beneath your palm as you hold its tiny body in your hand. It will open its eyes and look at you. However, this is seldom the case. If it happens to you, it is one of the hardest things anyone can endure. Don't let the possibility of a fetal demise ruin your pregnancy, but know that it is something that can happen. If it does happen, don't beat yourself up for it. Don't think that there had to be a sign, somewhere, that you could have seen if *only* you'd been paying attention. That isn't always the case.

You can try doing kick counts—count the number of times your baby is kicking per hour. If it kicks less than 10 times in an hour, call your doctor. If you are feeling contractions and you are still in early-to-mid pregnancy, call your doctor. If you smoke or do drugs, quit—as using these products can increase your risk of a stillbirth and let your doctor know.

After the birth of your stillborn baby, the doctors can do certain tests to find out if they can figure out why the baby died. They will run blood tests to check for genetic disorders. They will ask if you want an autopsy. They may even ask for a drug test. The results could help you understand why your baby died, and help stop it from happening in the future. However, sometimes no reason can be found. Sometimes the baby just died or stopped growing and no one can tell you why. Sometimes, I think, that is the worst part—the not knowing why. You can rail and yell and be angry, but you have nothing to direct it towards. If you knew it was because of a certain *thing*, a certain *reason*, you'd know what to blame.

Once you have a stillborn baby, you are at higher risk of having another. It is completely up to you on when and if you are going to try again. Your caregiver will more than likely suggest you wait at least three months before trying again, to not only give your body time to heal, but to also give your heart time to heal.

Your chances of having a stillborn are higher if

You are over 35

You are obese

You smoke tobacco or drink alcohol

You take drugs

You've had previous stillbirths

You've taken pain medications during pregnancy

You have high blood pressure

You have liver disease

You have a history of blood clots

You have a multiple pregnancy (more than one baby)

You are African-American

Your baby is not growing

You have been in an accident, fallen, or are physically abused

Let your caregiver know if you have any of these risk factors.

What is Preeclampsia?

Preeclampsia can typically start after the 20th week. Preeclampsia affects the baby's placenta and the mother's kidneys. It is usually signified by a sudden change in blood pressure; your blood pressure is higher than normal. If seizures start, it has turned into Eclampsia, which is one of the leading causes of maternal death in the United States. There is no known cause for preeclampsia and the only way to cure it is by delivering the baby. If your preeclampsia is severe or if it develops into full blown Eclampsia, your caregiver will induce or perform a C-section even if you are not near your due date. They do this to save your life, but also to try to save the baby's life, if possible. Preeclampsia can

Prevent the baby's placenta from giving the baby nutrients through the blood—they don't get enough;

Cause the placenta to calcify;

Lead to premature birth

Turn into Eclampsia, which can lead to seizure, coma, and maternal death.

What Are the Signs of Preeclampsia?

There are signs that your doctor will look for to determine if you have preeclampsia. The caregiver will look for these signs of preeclampsia

High blood pressure

Protein in the urine

Rapid swelling in extremities

Rapid weight gain

Dizziness

Seeing spots

Faintness

Nausea and vomiting

Severe headaches

If you have these signs, your caregiver will usually prescribe complete or partial bed rest. In bad cases, the caregiver will have you stay in the hospital for close observation. This is to give the baby time to develop, so if your condition worsens, the baby has a higher chance at living if you need to be delivered early. Your caregiver may prescribe medications to manage the condition, and if you are close to your due date, they may just opt to induce.

Other Complications to Watch For

Sadly, pregnancy isn't a wonderland of awesomeness for all women and complications do arise. You can't stop everything bad from happening and not everything can be foreseen. Some of the complications that can happen during a normal, healthy pregnancy are preterm labor, placental abruption, gallstones, low amniotic fluid, and placenta previa.

Preterm labor is labor that develops before the 37th week of pregnancy. If you start having regular contractions before you are 37 weeks pregnant, and they are causing your cervix to dilate and efface, you may be in premature labor. You may be going into premature labor if

you have four or more contractions in one hour or you have painful, period-like cramps

your discharge changes—becomes more watery, mucous-like, or bloody you have pressure in your pelvic area that is more intense than normal

you have a dull, rhythmic back pain

you are bleeding

your water breaks

If you experience any of these symptoms, call your caregiver right away or head to the nearest emergency room.

Preterm labor can generally be slowed at the hospital, and many women who go into preterm labor can go on to have their babies after the 37th week of pregnancy.

Placental abruption is when your placenta starts to tear away from your uterine wall before you have given birth, and it can be dangerous for both the mother and the baby. Symptoms are

vaginal bleeding which can happen very rapidly, or develop slowly, it can be pink to deep red;

abdominal pain and uterine tenderness,

back pain,

rapid contractions with no rest between.

If you have any of these symptoms call your caregiver right away. It isn't possible to reattach a placenta that has torn away from the uterine wall, but with the right care you could still go on to give birth to a healthy baby. Your caregiver will more than likely hospitalize you for close observation, and in some cases, they will give you steroids to help your baby's lungs mature. If the bleeding stops and your baby is fine, your caregiver may let you stay on bed rest at home. The bed rest is meant to stop your placenta from tearing more, and it's essential that you follow your caregiver's instructions. If you are close to term, your caregiver may opt to deliver the baby, either via induction or C-section, depending on the severity of the abruption.

Gallstones are stones that form in your gallbladder and can cause pain when they emerge from your gallbladder and become stuck on their way out. They can obstruct the liver, and cause bile to overflow into your stomach. Unfortunately, women are more prone to gallstones during pregnancy. The symptoms for gallstones are

severe pain in the upper part of your abdomen or between your shoulder blades (it isn't the same for everyone)

indigestion and nausea (worse than normal)

dark, orange or neon yellow urine or light colored stool

skin or white of eyes turning yellow

The type of care you receive for gallstones depends on how severe your gallstones are (the caregiver can order an ultrasound to find out how extent the problem is) and how far along you are in your pregnancy. The caregiver may prescribe medication and pain pills for the gallstone attacks. If you are in your second trimester, they may opt to remove your gallbladder, as surgery is safest in the second trimester. However, if the condition can be managed by diet and/or medication, the caregiver will more than likely wait until after you have given birth to perform the surgery. You can avoid gallstones by eating a diet low in fatty and fried foods.

Low amniotic fluid is when you do not have enough amniotic fluid in your uterus to support your baby's growth. At each appointment, your caregiver will measure your uterus for growth. If your caregiver finds that there is little or no growth, they will schedule or perform an ultrasound that will check your fluid levels. If it is low, they will closely monitor your pregnancy to ensure your baby is growing normally via ultrasounds, biophysical profiles, and non-stress tests. If you are near term or the baby is not thriving inside the womb, your caregiver will either induce you or perform a C-section.

Placenta previa is generally diagnosed early in pregnancy or at the 20th week ultrasound appointment. The placenta can attach to the uterine wall in any position; it can be anterior or posterior, either near the front of the uterus or the back of the uterus respectively. However, sometimes it can attach in such a way that it is entirely covering your cervix; this is called placenta previa. If it is entirely covering your cervix, you will not be allowed to birth the baby naturally; your caregiver will perform a C-section. However, most (not all) women who have been diagnosed with placenta previa go on to have a normal delivery, because the placenta can move away from the cervix as the baby grows. Your doctor will keep a careful eye on your placenta before allowing you to go into labor naturally.

Chapter 13: The Baby inside You

What does a Baby Look Like inside the Womb?

Your baby changes rapidly during the first trimester, and while it is forming, especially at the beginning, it does not look much like a baby. However, the little cells are working hard, creating fingers, toes, organs, bone structure, and brain parts.

The First Trimester: During the first trimester it goes from the size of a poppy seed all the way up to the size of a plum. It's hard to imagine anything growing that fast! You're going through changes as well as the hormones surge through your body. You may find yourself nauseous often, and you may be visited by vomiting. You may start to feel more tired than usual. Take extra naps and enjoy the extra sleep. Sleep will be a distant memory soon.

- Week 5: This is usually how far along you are before you find out you are pregnant, and your little one is the size of an apple seed. At this stage, it is still an embryo and it looks a bit like a tadpole. The major organs are starting to form, as well as the nervous, digestive, and circulatory systems. That little embryo is busy!

- Week 6: By now, your baby is the size of a pea, approximately a quarter of an inch long. Its facial features are starting to form. Its heart is beating rapidly and blood is starting to circulate. The fingers and toes are formed and are webbed.

- Week 7: Your little one is about a half an inch long already. Twice its size in one week! The brain is on the fast track and generates about one hundred new cells every single minute! The kidneys are in place and its little legs and arms start to emerge.

- Week 8: Your baby is already moving all over the place, though you probably can't feel it. The webbing is starting to disappear from the fingers and toes and her taste buds are forming.

- Week 9: Not only is your baby the size of an olive, but it also has a new name—fetus! Her facial features are developing rapidly and if you are lucky, you may be able to hear the heartbeat at this appointment.

- Week 10: Your baby is now over an inch long. Her joints are working and her little bones and cartilage are forming furiously. Her fingernails and hair are starting to grow. She's not only moving more and kicking, but she is practicing swallowing.

- Week 11: Your baby is over an inch and a half long and a quarter of an ounce. She's lost most of her tadpole look and looks more like a baby already. The webbing around her fingers and toes is completely gone.

- Week 12: Your baby is now the size of a plum. She's over two inches long and nearly a half an ounce. Most of her systems are fully formed and are growing rapidly. She's developing reflexes, opening and closing her fingers, and developing her brain.

The Second Trimester: Your hormone levels are dropping, and usually that means less nausea. The fatigue you've been fighting with for the last twelve weeks reduces, and you'll find yourself with more energy. You may even look pregnant now.

- Week 13: She's measuring in at nearly three inches. Her teeth are starting to form (below the gum line) and her vocal cords are forming. Her intestines are moving into place and her tiny fingers already have fingerprints.

- Week 14: Your baby weighs one and a half ounces and measures over three inches long. He sure has been busy! He may already be sucking his thumb. His kidneys, liver, and spleen are working hard. Thin, fuzz-like hair called lanugo is starting to grow all over his body.

- Week 15: Your baby has gained an entire ounce in one week and measures at about four inches. He's moving all over the place; you may or may not feel the movement yet. He may also be hiccupping already, and all his joints and limbs are on the move.

- Week 16: Oh how she's grown. She's now the size of an avocado, measuring a bit over four and a half inches and weighing about three and a half ounces. Her hair, including brows and lashes, are growing in more rapidly. She can hear your voice.

- Week 17: He's now over five inches and is five ounces in weight. All that cartilage is starting to turn to bone and he's starting to put on weight.

- Week 18: The baby is about the size of a sweet potato. He yawns, hiccups, sucks, and swallows. His punches and kicks may be able to be felt now. An ultrasound at this time may be able to indicate gender.

- Week 19: Baby has become roughly the size of a mango, measuring six inches and weighing over eight ounces. She is starting to form her vernix, which is a greasy, white film that covers her entire body. She'll still have some of this on her at birth, but it wipes right off. It's a skin protectant and helps keep her comfy inside your womb. Her brain is developing the five senses.

- Week 20: Your baby has sure grown! Her taste buds are now working. She's kicking like crazy and you may feel it for the first time this week. You will probably get an ultrasound this week to check for baby's growth and health. If you are lucky, and if you want to know, they may be able to see the gender if the baby cooperates.

- Week 21: She's ten and a half inches long now, and weighs approximately twelve ounces. Her digestive system is making meconium (the first poop she makes in her diaper, which is black, sticky, and tarlike). If it is a girl, her eggs are already formed—the whole lifetime supply of them.

- Week 22: She is starting to take up a lot of room. You may notice a stretch mark or two around this time, and if you're skinny, your belly button may start to pop out. While you are becoming increasingly uncomfortable, she's snuggling down for a nice sleep and does so in cycles.

- Week 23: This is the time the "average" baby really starts to range in size and weight. Your baby is nearly a foot long and weighs anywhere from twelve to twenty ounces. She's fully formed and really starting to put on weight. She's listening to your heartbeat, but also to other outside sounds.

- Week 24: She's roughly the size of a grapefruit now. Your doctor may order a glucose test this week. You are feeling more and more movement from your little one. Her capillaries have recently formed, giving her translucent skin a more natural, human look.

- Week 25: Your baby is now over a foot long and can measure anywhere from one and a half to two and a half pounds. She knows which way is up and which way is down. She's gaining weight and her hair may be getting longer.

- Week 26: Her eyelashes have grown in and soon she will be able to open her eyes. Her immune system is ramping up for life on the outside and she's starting to practice breathing. She's not breathing air; her lungs are full of amniotic fluid. However, these practice breaths strengthen her lungs and give her good practice.

- Week 27: She's still gaining weight rapidly and her lungs are getting stronger. She is now showing brain activity—she's thinking and perhaps dreaming. Ultrasounds may show more thumb sucking. Also, if you are thinking about scheduling a 3d ultrasound, now is the time to make your appointment. The pictures turn out better from weeks 27 to 30.

The Third Trimester: You're almost there and so is she! You may be sleeping less due to discomfort and find yourself getting up often at night. If you can't sleep, find something that helps you relax. Your breasts already have colostrum in them (the food your baby eats before your milk comes in) and you may start feeling Braxton Hicks contractions. These contractions are generally not painful and help tone the uterus for delivery.

- Week 28: She's about the size of an eggplant, can still weigh anywhere from one and half to two and a half pounds and measure anywhere from thirteen and a half inches to a little over fourteen inches. She's getting fatter and her skin is losing its wrinkly look. Her lungs are mature and if you were to go into labor, she may survive now. As each week passes, her chances are higher.

- Week 29: Your baby is topping the charts at fifteen to sixteen inches long and two and a half to three and a half pounds. He is moving like crazy because his energy is up—he's growing white fat deposits. You may even begin to feel him hiccupping.

- Week 30: Your baby is now as long as a cucumber. And while his skin is growing smoother, his brain is getting curvier; wrinkles are forming in his brain to keep up with his brain development. He can now grasp with his hands and ultrasounds may show him holding his hands or playing with his umbilical cord!

- Week 31: Your baby may now measure sixteen inches long and weigh up to three and a half (or more) pounds. The irises in his eyes can now react to light and his five senses are now all working.

- Week 32: She's probably turned head down by now but don't let it bother you if she hasn't; there is plenty of time. You both may be feeling like you're running out of room in there.

- Week 33: Your baby now weighs around four to five pounds and could be seventeen to eighteen inches long. Her eyes are open now when she's awake, and breathing, sucking, and swallowing are now more coordinated. Her bones are stronger as well.

- Week 34: He's just about the size of a butternut squash. He recognizes and reacts to your voice and even to songs you sing. He is urinating about two cups worth a day. His urine is part of the amniotic fluid, which cycles through your little one's body daily.

- Week 35: She won't grow in length much from here on out, but she'll continue gaining weight. She'll gain about a half a pound each week. If you're having a boy, his testes are more than likely fully descended by now.

- Week 36: If you haven't bought a car seat yet, now would be the time to get one. If you have one, install it. If baby were born now, he'd more than likely be fine. If not, he may need extra care at the hospital. If you haven't created a birth plan yet, now would be the time to do it. You need to give a copy to your caregiver for your records and be sure he or she is OK with your birth plan. The baby is all geared up to come out and may have turned head down and descended a bit to give you more breathing room. He may not have yet—don't worry, some babies wait until you go into labor to get into place. Most of his critical systems are in excellent working order.

- Week 37: Your baby has reached full term! She is the size she is meant to be (but will still gain weight every week she is in the womb). If you go into labor now, your caregiver will not try to stop you. Your baby is continuing to practice her breathing and is getting ready for her first diaper load.

- Week 38: Baby can be anywhere from fifteen to twenty-two inches long, and somewhere over six pounds; it all depends on how you grow babies. His hair maybe an inch long (or less, some babies are born with a head full, and some are born with fuzz), and he's starting to shed his vernix.

- Week 39: Your baby is still growing in weight and could be the size of a watermelon now. You will sure feel like he is as your belly feels like one. He can flex his joints, and his fingernails are maybe peaking over his fingertips. Every week he gains weight and grows smarter, so every week you keep him in, the more prepared he'll be for the world.

- Week 40: Even if you were to get an ultrasound today, it could be off by at least two pounds, so if your doctor tells you the baby weighs *this much*, keep that in mind. You may go into labor soon, but you may not. A first time pregnancy normally lasts until 41 weeks and five days.

- Weeks 41 – 43: Hopefully you will have had your baby by now, but if not, your doctor may discuss induction with you. The baby is fully grown and now able to live outside of your womb. Also, your placenta can start to deteriorate after time and leave your baby without nutrients. Most babies will emerge on their own at the end of the 42nd week, and if your caregiver allows you to remain pregnant that long, your baby will be born healthy. You are probably more than ready for baby to come out, however, and may find the idea of induction hard to resist.

Can You Reduce Birth Defects?

The causes of many types of birth defects are unknown, though there are some things you can do to try to prevent some.

- See your doctor for your regular prenatal appointments.

- Make a pre-conception appointment to find out if you, or the father, are at risk for any genetic disorders.

- Take enough folic acid both before pregnancy and during pregnancy to prevent neural tube defects like spina bifida.

- Stop drinking, smoking and taking drugs. All of these are known to cause birth defects.

- Check with your caregiver about the medication you are taking; some medications have been known to cause birth defects.

- Make sure your vaccinations are all up-to-date before getting pregnant.

- Avoid harmful substances: paint thinners, pesticides, lead-based paints, and contaminated water, to name a few.

While these steps can't prevent all birth defects, they are steps in the right direction.

Caution: What You Take May Harm Your Baby

When people think about substances that can harm their baby, they often think of street drugs, cigarettes, or alcohol. Many people do not realize that the drugs they are prescribed by their doctors could harm their baby. That is why it is important to talk to your doctor about your medications before you conceive or as soon as you conceive. Many antidepressants have not been tested on pregnant women, but have been shown to cause birth defects in rats.

Sometimes, doctors don't realize how a drug will affect the fetus until it's too late, so find out if there is a natural alternative or if you are OK to go without the drug for nine months.

Some common drugs to avoid during pregnancy include such things as ibuprofen, naproxen, and aspirin. Ibuprofen, which is the main ingredient in Advil and Motrin, and naproxen, which is the main ingredient in Aleve, decreases the blood flow to the baby. Aspirin thins the blood and can lead to bleeding problems for both of you. If you have indigestion, don't take PeptoBismol, but ask your doctor about alternatives. If you get a cold, avoid any product that contains guaifenesin, which can increase the risk of neural tube defects; this is commonly found in products like Mucinex and Robitussin. That is why it is important to tell your caregiver about every medication you are taking, prescription or otherwise.

Even certain teas can have an adverse effect on your pregnancy. Some green teas contain caffeine, which does cross the placenta. Some herbal teas can be unsafe as well. Always talk to your caregiver about any concerns you have.

How to Ensure Healthy Brain Development of Your Baby during Pregnancy

The best way to ensure your baby's brain starts healthy and stays healthy is to avoid any medications that cause neural tube defects, stop smoking, stop drinking, stop taking street drugs, and by taking folic acid. You can also encourage baby's brain to continue growing stronger by eating healthy and taking fish oil (DHA) supplements. Avoiding stress will also help as well.

Why Do Babies Kick Inside the Womb?

The term "kicking" doesn't really cover what a baby does inside the womb. Baby moves his arms or legs, rolls, moves his head, and bends arms and knees. This is in preparation for life on the outside. Consider the movements people make to tone their muscles. They bend their knees, twist their torsos, raise and lower their arms—this is exactly what baby is doing. These movements are just the beginning to a healthy, strong baby.

The movement actually starts as early as four to five weeks, but you won't be able to feel it until much later. The baby is too small and too far inside your tummy for you to feel it. Some women can feel movement as early as 13 weeks, while others don't feel anything until 25 weeks. Feeling baby move for the first time is generally referred to as quickening, and it is one of the most wonderful feelings a pregnant woman experiences. Every movement is a reminder that you are creating life. It's a touch from baby to mother; a moment that remains special and sacred to you throughout your pregnancy. Sharing the feeling with your partner isn't easy at first, as it is only felt from the inside. Enjoy this time with your baby. It means he is healthy and strong and is just getting stronger.

Chapter 14: Pre-Delivery: What You Need to Know?

Why Would a Childbirth Class Be Helpful?

Childbirth classes can educate you about your impending delivery, teach relaxation techniques, and give you important information about which types of pain relief are available for you at your hospital. Which type of class you take depends on what type of birth you want to have. If you are delivering at a hospital, you will more than likely end up using some sort of pain relief; childbirth classes give you the knowledge you need to choose the best option for yourself. Even if you are planning on having a natural birth, that is a drug-free birth, it is good to understand your options if things get too intense. Some women will opt for pain relieving drugs without understanding what possible side-effects that drug may have on them or the baby. This is when a childbirth class could help you determine which side-effects you are willing to expose yourself to if the pain becomes too intense. However, there are many different types of childbirth classes available to you, both through your hospital and out of pocket.

What Types of Childbirth Classes Are There?

Some insurances pay for childbirth classes through your doctor's office or through the hospital. If you don't want to have a high out-of-pocket expense, this may be the best way for you to go. Find out what your hospital offers and whether or not your insurance will cover the costs of the classes. If you have enough money to pay for out-of-pocket classes, however, then you can be a bit choosier. When looking for a class, find out if the class is in line with your expectations for delivery. If it is an in-person class (versus online or self-study) find out what the teacher's credentials or experience are, and how many couples are going to be taking the class with you. Location is another factor for consideration, as well as the time the classes meet. It won't do you much good to schedule a childbirth class that is thirty minutes away and starts ten minutes after work.

Lamaze classes: Lamaze classes don't only teach you breathing and relaxation techniques, but they also teach you about normal births, medications, breastfeeding, C-sections, and basic labor techniques. Most Lamaze classes are at least twelve hours total. See www.lamazeinternational.org for more information regarding Lamaze Childbirth classes.

The Bradley Method or American Academy of Husband Coached Childbirth: The Bradley Method teaches childbirth as a natural human process. They teach you about natural birthing techniques and give you the knowledge to be a self-advocate. The Bradley Method emphasizes relaxation and natural birth and the course takes about twelve weeks to complete, so don't wait too long to schedule your classes. For more information on the Bradley Method, visit their website at www.bradleybirth.com.

International Childbirth Education Association: These are instructors who are taught through ICEA, and are usually the type of education courses available through hospitals or doctors' offices. They teach labor skills, comfort, medications, and possible complications. To learn more about the ICEA childbirth classes, or to find an instructor near you, visit www.icea.org.

Hypnobabies: Hypnobabies is class that can be taken in person or as a self-study home course. The cost is typically out-of-pocket and the self-study kit can be purchased through their website or through Amazon.com. This class is intended for natural, medication-free birthing, and can be used at home, at a birthing center, or in a hospital environment. It teaches you about your body during pregnancy, labor, and beyond. It gives you techniques to focus on during labor with an overarching goal of helping you achieve a pain-free, drug-free, calm birthing experience. You can find out more about it at www.hypnobabies.com. There are other self-hypnosis birthing classes out there, but this one takes a closer look at the body and gives you skills that you can use throughout your pregnancy and beyond. It is especially helpful if you are intent upon a drug-free birth.

There are many types of childbirth classes and not all of them have been covered here. What classes are available to you have a lot to do with what is available in your area. Find out what your local hospital offers and what is available in your region.

Why You Should Avoid Unnecessary Medical Interventions

First of all, what are unnecessary medical interventions? What these are may differ from person to person. For instance, I find fetal monitoring, Pitocin, and IVs to be unnecessary during childbirth. Hospitals, and most doctors, assume that childbirth is like a disease and treat it as such. You are heavily monitored. In some places, you are not allowed to consume food or water during labor. You are given an IV with saline solution to keep you hydrated instead. You are forced to remain immobile, usually on your back, and not allowed to move and rock, in some instances. Childbirth doesn't have to be painful, but when coupled with these interventions, it often is. Without food and water, your body quickly runs out of energy. Without the assistance of gravity, some babies have a hard time descending. Without the ability to move into a more comfortable position, the pain can become too intense. All of which can lead to pain medications, which often have the effect of lowering blood pressure and slowing down labor. Some medications have adverse effects upon people, and many women who get them find themselves shaking uncontrollably, vomiting or passing out. These drugs can also lead to Pitocin-induced contractions, which are not natural and are some of the most painful contractions. Often, the pain medications side-effects lead to C-sections, suction, forceps, or forced-pushing before the mother's body is completely ready to push.

Another medical intervention that is unnecessary in most cases is the artificial rupture of membranes (AROM). This is a technique doctors use to get labor going stronger. They insert a long stick-like instrument with a slight hook at the end into your vagina and up through your cervix. They hook this over your membranes and tug. This allows your water to break, which can intensify contractions and make them stronger. However, this also puts you and baby on a timeline. Once the waters are broken, doctors generally give you twelve hours to have the baby. If they feel you are not laboring fast enough or if labor has stalled, they will use Pitocin to further help your labor progress. Many problems can arise due to AROM. Once your water is broken, it is easier for bacteria to be introduced into your uterus. This is why you are put on a schedule. They are afraid of infections, both for you and the baby. However, what they have done by performing AROM is this: they have taken away the cushion that helped absorb the shock of the contractions. If your labor doesn't progress fast enough, they will give you Pitocin, which will make the contractions that much stronger, and generally will lead you to decide to use drugs or an epidural.

The epidural is supposed to numb you from the waist down. The anesthesiologist places a needle in between your vertebrae into your spinal cord. They do this while you are contracting, you will be asked to sit up and curl over your stomach while they try to insert the needle. This is not comfortable during a contraction at all. Then, a catheter is placed over the needle and through the hole into your spine. This catheter will deliver a drug into your spinal column, which deadens the sensation from the puncture all the way down to your toes. There are usually multiple drugs in this mixture, and you are often given a button you can push once every fifteen minutes to administer doses as needed. There are two types of epidurals given, the regular epidural and the "walking" epidural, though the latter name is a misnomer, as you are not allowed to walk anywhere once it is in place. There are side effects to all drugs, and the epidural is no exception. One of the most common side effects is a change in blood pressure. Another is a slowed down labor. Most women are told to push when they are at ten centimeters dilated, and when you have an epidural, you often cannot figure out how to push. This forced pushing can last for hours. If it goes on too long, the doctor may opt to perform a C-section, or use forceps or suction.

Another unnecessary medical intervention that is pretty outdated is the episiotomy. Most doctors no longer perform episiotomies, but some still do. An episiotomy is a procedure in which the doctor will cut your perineum prior to delivering the baby's head. This is a cut that goes from the bottom of your vaginal opening towards your anus. It is a painful cut and often takes longer to heal than a tear. It also remains painful longer than a tear does. In the past, doctors believed that a cleaner cut was a better choice; it was easier to clean and sew up. However, if you take a natural plant fiber and tear it, you will notice how easily the ends come together. If you wet it a bit, it looks like new. Now take that same fiber and cut it in a straight line using scissors. Do the ends come together more easily? No, and they will not stick together when wetted. Skin is much the same. Simple tears heal better than cuts. This being said, sometimes an episiotomy can mean the difference between tearing *up* your vagina or having a straight cut down. It should never be something that is done arbitrarily.

Sadly, many of these interventions have become so routinely used in a hospital environment that most nurses and doctors haven't seen a natural, medication-free birth in their entire careers. These medical interventions have a waterfall effect. Once you get the IV, asking for pain medication is easier. It is also easier for the doctors to administer Pitocin. Once the Pitocin is in place, it is almost a necessity to use pain medication, though some few women have worked through Pitocin-induced contractions without drugs. Pitocin can over stimulate your uterus and cause distress in the baby. You will not be able to walk around once you are on Pitocin, because you will need continual fetal monitoring, and a lot of times, movement can cause the monitor to slip and "lose" the baby's heartbeat, which scares the nursing staff. Once you are in place and unable to move, the contractions are more painful. If labor is long, and you are hungry, tired, and thirsty, it is easier to ask for medications. Medications have side effects and can affect both you and the baby. This is why childbirth classes are important. If you want a healthy pregnancy with a healthy result, it is important that you educate yourself on the effects of the routine drugs used during birth and decide if you'd want to risk those effects for you and your child. If you are able to have a natural, drug-free labor, it will be because you said no to many unnecessary medical interventions.

How to Create a Birth Plan to Avoid Unnecessary Medical Interventions

Birth plans are something you are usually taught about in childbirth education courses and can be very helpful when the big day comes. Create your birth plan when you are closer to your due date—I usually create mine around week 35. There are forms online you can download and use or you can create your own. There are no set rules to birth plans. Get together with your birth partner and create it together. This is not only a special bonding time between you two, but it is also a contract between you, your partner, and your doctor. When your partner helps you create one, they will know what your wishes are when the day comes, and it will enable them to be your advocate when you are not able to. The birth plan should have three essential sections:

Introduction:

- What your names are: yours, baby's (if known), and daddy's

- What type of birth you want (natural or medicated)

- What type of drugs you want if you are opting for medication

- Whether you want a heplock (the IV needle is inserted, but not hooked up to an IV bag) or the full IV.

- Whether you plan on eating and drinking or not

- What type of environment you want (quiet and dark, music or none...)

- Who will be in the room during certain times

Labor:

- What you are going to do during labor (for instance, if you are using hypnobabies, you would put here that you will not discuss pain, drugs, or use the terms, "labor, contractions, pain, or delivery")

- What drugs you will use if you are willing to use pain medication

- What positions you want to labor in—the ability to walk around, use a birthing ball, sit in a tub, etc...

- Whether or not students are allowed in your room (many hospitals are learning hospitals)

- Whether or not you want your water broke (No AROM, for example)

Delivery and after Delivery:

- How you want to deliver the baby (squat bar, break down bed, on your side, on your hands and knees)

- How you want to hold the baby after birth

For example: after pushing baby out, the mother would like to hold the baby using skin-on-skin contact on her chest.

- How and when you would like the cord to be cut

- Whether you will be getting the baby circumcised or not

- How you will be feeding the baby

- Whether you want a pacifier introduced or not

- What you want to do if the baby has problems (if the baby needs to be taken out of the room, the mother would like _____ to join him/her.)

- How early you want to leave the hospital

Once you have finished your birth plan, ask your doctor to look it over and have a signature area on the plan for you, your partner and your doctor to sign. You should make a copy for your medical chart, but also bring one with you to the hospital. If you are planning to breastfeed, you can also make signs to place on the baby's bassinet that says, "Breastfed baby, please do not give formula or pacifier." There are many things you may want to include on your birth plan that were not listed here and that's fine, this was not an extensive list.

Keep in mind, however, that nurses change shifts every twelve hours, so you will need to point out your birth plan as each new nurse arrives. Some nurses are laid back and understanding, while others do not want to hear about birth plans or argue about the way they do things. If you are not comfortable with your nurse, let someone know—she can easily be reassigned. Your comfort is paramount, after all. Discomfort and stress slow down labor.

What to Buy for Your Baby: The Essentials

Baby really doesn't need as many things as the stores and corporations say they do, but first time parents often go all out and buy everything on the market. What you need for your baby depends on where you live, how you live, what kind of parenting style you are going to have, and what you find essential. For instance, if you walk a lot, a stroller or a sling would be a great buy. If you spend a great deal of time in the car, then the stroller wouldn't get a lot of use. Also, you don't have to pay $450 dollars for a good stroller. Some of the best strollers I've had were under $50.

Essentials for breastfeeding:

- Lanolin for your nipples

- Breast pads

- Breast pump (if you are going to bottle feed/store milk)

- Milk storage bags (for freezing milk)

- Lactation consults or classes (Women, Infants, Children (WIC) offers breastfeeding essentials, and many can lend out or give you items you need. You should also look for your local La Leche League for women who can help you.)

- Time—the first two weeks of breastfeeding are the hardest. Once you get over that hump, the rest is usually cake.

Essentials for bottle feeding:

- Bottles

- Nipples

- Bottle brush

- Formula (can be expensive, breastfeeding is cheaper)

- Clean water

Don't use tap water or the microwave for a newborn's bottle. Warm tap water can contain contaminants and microwaves don't heat uniformly. Your baby can be burnt by a "hot spot" in the microwaved bottle.

Other supplies for home (nonessential):

- Bottle warmer (helpful for warming up cold formula or frozen breast milk)

- Baby wipe warmer

- Diaper pail (a regular garbage can will do)

- Changing station (any safe, flat surface will suffice)

- Crib (baby spends less time in the crib as a newborn than you are shown on TV. A simple bassinet or Moses basket works well.)

- Baby bathtub

- Baby lotions and shampoos

- Baby swing (though these can be life savers, they are not a necessity)

For care of the cord:

- Water

- Cotton balls or swabs

- Diapers that don't rub/cover the cord

For baby:

- Onesies—these pieces of clothing are the best and most-used pieces your newborn will wear. Other clothing is cute, but the frilly bits get in the way, aren't comfortable, and can't be slept in.

- One piece pajamas

- Blankets

- Burping cloths

- Diapers (either disposable or washable, depending on your preference)

- Baby wipes

- Pacifier (if you are using one)

- Car seat (this is necessary; you cannot even bring baby home from the hospital without one)

- Soft towels and wash cloths

There are more things that people buy for their baby, and this is just a small list compared to what a lot of people buy.

What You Should Bring to the Hospital or Birthing Center

What you bring to the hospital or birthing center is completely up to you. You can bring all things listed or none of the things listed. Most hospitals provide clothing (gowns) for you to wear during labor and delivery, but some women choose to wear their own clothes. What you need also depends on how long your stay will be and what type of birth it is. You may need different items if you are getting a C-section. This list is primarily for normal delivery.

- Camera, either still or video. If you plan on videotaping the birth, find out what the hospital policies are regarding videotaping during certain procedures. A camera is a must for most new parents. It's used to document the labor, birth, and the new baby on its first day of life. Make sure the batteries are charged and bring the charger!

- Makeup. Many women feel the need to put on makeup before getting their pictures taken. They want to look cute for the camera, which is usually impossible during labor. But also take it if you want to put it on before you leave the hospital. Maybe not your whole arsenal of cosmetics, but some lip gloss, mascara, and eye shadow may come in handy.

- Robe or pajamas: Some women refuse to wear hospital gowns and would rather use their own clothes either during labor, after labor, or both. I prefer to use the gown during labor and then to change into comfortable pajamas when it is all over. The robe can be helpful if you are able to walk around the hospital and you don't want your bottom to peek out of your gown at everyone you pass. However, if you don't have one or forget one, you can use another gown as a robe—just put it on backwards.

- Socks. The hospital will give you slipper socks to wear, which is nice if your water breaks, because then they just throw them away. You won't have to bundle up your own and put them back in your bag all wet and nasty. You can still bring some though for after the birth.

- Slippers/Sandals. These are nice to have if you are walking around the hospital and don't want to step in anything while wearing just socks. Find some with good traction, though; hospital floors are slick!

- Take home outfit for baby. I always bring a couple of different outfits in different sizes. I always have a preemie set on hand, as well as a normal "newborn" size. This is because my babies are often on the smaller size and newborn clothes are too big.

Find something that is cute and can be kept as a sort of family heirloom.

- Baby blanket. Hospitals used to give you the baby blanket you had your baby wrapped in at the hospital, but no more. You must bring your own baby blankets, so your baby can be covered from the elements on the way out of the hospital.

- Car seat. Most hospitals won't allow you to leave until you bring the car seat up to your room and strap the baby in. The nurse will check to be sure the baby fits inside the seat correctly. Don't use car seat covers or seat belt covers unless they come with the car seat, however, because most car seats are not tested with these additional add-ons (unless they come with them). You can use bundled up baby blankets around baby (but not under the seat belts) if the car seat is a bit too roomy.

- Toiletries. Bring toothbrushes and toothpaste for everyone. Shampoo and conditioner are not provided by the hospital, either. You may want to bring your own washcloths. If you do, make sure they are not white. Bring your own pads for the ride home. The hospital often uses disposable diapers for postpartum pads.

- Money and/or food from home. You may not need money to call mom and dad anymore, but you may want to visit the snack machine in the middle of the night. Often mom is fed, but dad is left to fend for himself. Also, babies don't understand time and like to come out whenever they want. They don't care if the cafeteria is open or not, and you will be starving after you've given birth, even if you've eaten through labor. Most hospital rooms have little refrigerators for your personal food and drinks. If yours doesn't, ask the nursing staff if you can store it in the kitchen (most have one for patients).

- Clothes to go home in. These are a change of clothes for you, though most new moms leave the hospital wearing the clothes they came in with. Include a nursing bra and nursing pads. The washable ones are the best.

- Massage tools. You may want your birth partner to massage your back, your shoulders, or your feet (either during labor or after). Feel free to bring oils for this. A little pampering is nice after a long, hard day of working. If you want your partner to perform a perineal massage, bring a bit of olive oil for the perineum, or whatever oil you have been using at home.

- Music. You can bring your mp3 player or a CD. Most, but not all, hospitals have CD players you can use to listen to your own mood music. I bring my mp3 player. I am much more comfortable with it in my ears, than trying to listen to it over everyone's talking.

- Pillows. Feel free to bring your own pillows. Make sure the pillow cases are colored so they won't be mistaken for hospital property.

Pack a bag for daddy. Let's face it: there is only so much a man can do while you are working through your contractions. They can rub you, hold your hand, or "dance" with you, but sometimes you don't want to be touched. Plus, if you are being induced slowly, it can be an even more boring experience for him. Pack a book, some magazines, and maybe a handheld game or tablet for your poor spouse to play on while the time is slowly moving forward. Don't worry, when things start happening, he won't have time for all of that stuff. On the upside, if you bring a tablet or laptop, you can post status updates and pictures on the fly.

Pack extra clothes for dad. If you decide to get into the shower and want his help, a pair of swimming trunks will go a long way. Also, you will probably be staying overnight. Pack some night clothes for him and some clean clothes for the next day.

If you go into labor and you haven't packed your bag, don't worry. None of this stuff is *essential* and most of it can be picked up after delivery if you really want it. Even if you can't leave, most family members are happy to run errands for you if you need them to. The hospital will have everything you need for your stay. You can always make a list and give it to your husband after you have the baby.

What Items Are Needed for a Home Birth?

Most midwives will provide you with a list of things you need to have at home in order to have a home birth. Their lists may differ from mine—and that's fine! Follow your midwives' list; they know what they have on hand already.

- Plastic drop cloth or plastic sheet

- Cotton balls

- Bath towels and wash cloths (at least four each)

- Plastic trash bags

- Two fitted sheets and two flat sheets on your bed

- Receiving blankets (at least eight)

- Plastic mixing bowls: large and small

- Flashlight: working and with extra batteries

- Toilet paper

- Duct tape

- Thermometer with probe covers

- Diapers

- Pads (for you)

- Juice to drink

- Bag of ice

- Proteins to eat (peanut butter, eggs, cheese)

- Clothes ready for you and baby after birth

You may also rent a birthing tub. Your midwife will let you know what items you need to have on hand for the birth. She will ask you to have it all available at least three weeks before your due date. You will also need to be sure you have certain things in a separate paper bag that is marked as your birth kit, so you won't have to look all over for clothes and receiving blankets after you've given birth. Another thing you may want to do is make brownies or cookies to give to the midwife when she shows up. Make enough for her and her assistant.

Identify True Labor Contractions

Contractions are different depending on the woman and the position of the baby. Most start out feeling like menstrual cramps. The problem with quantifying a contraction is the fact that they can differ from pregnancy to pregnancy as well as from woman to woman. Usually the pain starts low and moves up. Sometimes it is a dull ache in the back or thighs. Sometimes, they feel like intense gas pains. The pain radiates from one point to the next—from the bottom of the uterus to the top or vice versa. One way to verify if it is a true contraction, and not Braxton Hicks, is to lie down, get in the shower or bath, walk around, and drink water. If the contractions stop or slow down during any of these activities, then they are not true labor contractions. True contractions do not stop or slow down when you move. True contractions come in intervals that are usually spaced apart for the same amount of time. For instance, contractions often start happening once every fifteen minutes. True labor gets stronger, more intense, and the contractions become more closely spaced.

Call your doctor if

- You have more than five contractions in an hour

- Your water has broken (sometimes it is a slow leak)

- You have bleeding

- You have intense pressure in your pelvic region or your vagina

Pay attention to the time if your water breaks; your caregiver will want to know when it occurred. Time your contractions and know how long they are and how far apart they are before you call your caregiver. He or she will let you know when to come into the hospital or birthing center, or let you know when they will arrive at your home to check up on you.

What to Expect during Delivery

While each birth is different, there are certain things you can expect during delivery. These expectations can change from woman to woman and from environment to environment; however, most women will encounter these experiences regardless of location.

Once you show up at the hospital, expect to be checked for dilation or amniotic fluid leaks, especially if your water has already broken. If you are checking in for an induction, delivery is much the same, except you may be on continuous fetal monitoring. You will more than likely not be allowed to eat, drink, or walk around the hospital.

Check-in: You will be taken into a room, which may be the room the baby will be birthed in, but it could be a triage room. The nurse will check your dilation and if you are at 3 centimeters or more, you will be allowed to check in. Most delivery rooms are private and you will remain in that room for the entirety of your stay. Some hospitals have separate labor and delivery rooms and will move you to a new room once you've had the baby. During this time, your nurses will review your birth plan, have you sign admittance paper work, a living will, and get your insurance information. If you are in active labor, though, they will wait to get most of this information. A heplock or an IV will also be placed now.

Labor: During labor, you will be given the chance to walk around the room and/or the hospital. Walking and rocking can help baby get into a better birthing position and help your cervix dilate and efface (soften). Your nurses will check your cervical position periodically, unless you have it on your birth plan that you don't want these checks. You may have to be put on a fetal monitor once every hour for fifteen minutes at a time. This is to check how your baby is doing during contractions. Some hospitals have jet tubs that you can sit in during labor, and this may help you manage the pain of contractions. However, they won't let you birth in the tub, so if you get close to delivering while in the bath, be prepared to stand up and walk out of the tub.

Delivery: You will be returned to your bed. If your birth plan includes birthing in different positions, your doctor may allow it. However, the doctors are much more interested in how much they can see, so may try to get you to lay back and put your legs up. Some doctors and nurses still have you hold your legs close to your body and push in a curling position. They may count down during the pushing phase to help you time how long you are pushing. You will know when it is time to push. I suggest you put something in your birth plan that argues for mother-led pushing, instead of doctor led pushing.

When you are about 7 to 8 centimeters dilated, you will go into transition. This is the final step your cervix takes to completely efface and dilate. Your contractions will last longer and be much closer together. This is the phase of labor in which most women "lose control" and want pain medication. It does not last long, but it is intense and powerful. Sometimes, you are given a short breather by your body after transition. Contractions will stop for a moment and you will have a little bit of time to pull yourself together. When contractions start again, they will feel different. You will feel more pressure in your vagina and your body will start pushing on its own. If your doctor hasn't arrived yet, you will be told to stop pushing. This is nearly impossible when your body is doing all of the work.

Mother-led pushing allows you to push when you feel like it; when it feels right. You will not need to be counted down or told when to push—you will know when and your body knows how. There is really very little pushing that needs to be done during this phase, as the baby is descending no matter how red your face gets. The hardest hurdle during this phase is to allow your muscles to relax while baby is descending and not to tense up. You may or may not feel a "ring of fire" as the baby's head passes through your vaginal opening. This is the final stretching of the area and it can also be pretty intense. After the head is out, most of the hard work is done. The doctor may ask you to stop pushing for a moment while they help the baby turn and make sure the umbilical cord is not in danger of being pinched, or if it is around the baby's neck, they will unwind it. The body usually slides out in a couple more pushes, depending on the size of the baby and how they are positioned.

After delivery: After you have delivered your baby, the baby will be placed with you for a bit and you may be allowed to breastfeed for a while. The baby will be placed on a warmer for a time where it will be measured and weighed, and its mouth and nose will be suctioned. Depending on your preferences, the baby will be given her first hepatitis B shot, a vitamin K shot, and eye drops. They will check the baby's blood sugar and make sure her breathing is good. If your baby is healthy, she will room-in with you during your stay at the hospital, unless you ask the nurses to take the baby to the nursery. Be aware, however, if you choose this option and are breastfeeding. The nurses may not want to wake you for a feeding and may supplement formula.

C-section: If you are coming in for a C-section, the expectations for after delivery are much the same as for any other birth. You will be asked to come in at a certain time. The doctor and nurses will check your vital signs, insert an epidural and make sure it is working as intended. You will be wheeled into a surgical suite. A tent-like structure will be erected above your abdomen so you won't have to watch the doctors at work. Your partner will usually sit up near your head. You should feel no pain, but you will feel tugging and pulling sensations as they maneuver your outer layers of muscle and fat to get to the baby. You will also feel tugging when they are taking the baby out. The baby will be taken directly to the warmer where it will be suctioned, weighed, tested, and monitored for a time while you are stitched up. You will be taken to a recovery room and the baby will be allowed to room-in with you if you wish. You will be able to nurse if you choose. Your stay will typically be longer after a C-section than it would be after a normal delivery, but only by a day or two if your recovery goes well.

www.ingramcontent.com/pod-product-compliance
Lightning Source LLC
Chambersburg PA
CBHW060202290526
45789CB00003B/1123